DEALING WITH CHRONIC KIDNEY DISEASE

A Guidebook on Identification, Treatment, and Management of CKD.

Joshua Kendall

TABLE OF CONTENTS

TABLE OF CONTENTS 2
1. INTRODUCTION TO CHRONIC KIDNEY DISEASE 3
    Understanding the Fundamentals 4
    Prevalence and Consequences 5
2: ANATOMY AND FUNCTION OF THE KIDNEYS 7
    Structure of the Kidneys 8
    Functions and Importance 11
3: DIAGNOSING CHRONIC KIDNEY DISEASE 17
    Screening Tests and Diagnostic Procedures 18
    Interpreting Test Results 22
    Identifying Underlying Causes 25
4: STAGES OF CHRONIC KIDNEY DISEASE 33
    Overview of CKD Stages: 34
    Progression and Monitoring 44
5: TREATMENT OPTIONS FOR CHRONIC KIDNEY
DISEASE 50
    Medications for Symptom Management 50
    Lifestyle Modifications for Kidney Health 61
    Dietary Adjustments for Kidney Disease 62
6: ADVANCED TREATMENT MODALITIES 73
    Hemodialysis and Peritoneal Dialysis 74
    Kidney Transplantation 77
    Palliative Care for End-Stage Kidney Disease 81
7: MANAGING COMPLICATIONS OF CHRONIC KIDNEY
DISEASE 87
    Hypertension and Cardiovascular Disease 88
    Anemia and Bone Disorders: 92

    Electrolyte Imbalance and Fluid Management.................96
8: LIVING WELL WITH CHRONIC KIDNEY DISEASE...105
    Coping Strategies and Emotional Support.....................105
    Maintaining Quality of Life 114
    Accessing Support Resources.......................................123
9: SPECIAL CONSIDERATIONS IN CHRONIC KIDNEY DISEASE..134
    CKD in Children and Adolescents 137
    CKD in Older Adults...145
    CKD and Pregnancy..153
10: FUTURE DIRECTIONS IN CHRONIC KIDNEY DISEASE MANAGEMENT...162
    Emerging Therapies and Technologies:........................163
    Promising Research Areas 171
    Advocacy and Community Engagement......................179
Vote of Thanks 190

1. INTRODUCTION TO CHRONIC KIDNEY DISEASE

Welcome to "Dealing With Chronic Kidney Disease: A Guidebook on Identification, Treatment, and Management of CKD." This comprehensive guide delves deeply into the multifaceted realm of Chronic Kidney Disease (CKD), offering a detailed examination of its intricate nuances, widespread prevalence, and profound implications for individuals and societies across the globe. Through meticulous exploration, we aim to illuminate the foundational elements of CKD, providing insight into its underlying mechanisms, epidemiological trends, and far-reaching consequences on health and well-being. By navigating through this extensive resource, readers will gain a comprehensive understanding of CKD's complex landscape, empowering them to navigate its challenges with informed awareness and proactive measures.

Understanding the Fundamentals

At the core of this comprehensive manual lies a commitment to unraveling the fundamental principles underpinning Chronic Kidney Disease (CKD). We embark on this journey by methodically simplifying the foundational elements, equipping readers with a robust understanding essential for navigating the complex landscape of kidney health. Through meticulous exploration, our aim is to not only define CKD but also delve deep into its intricate mechanisms and multifaceted risk factors. By furnishing readers with comprehensive insights and detailed analyses, our overarching objective is to empower individuals with the knowledge and comprehension necessary to make informed decisions regarding their health and overall well-being. Through this extensive resource, readers will embark on a transformative journey, gaining a profound understanding of CKD and its profound implications, thereby enabling them to navigate their health journey with confidence and clarity.

Prevalence and Consequences

Chronic Kidney Disease (CKD) stands as a formidable global health challenge, exerting far-reaching effects on individuals, families, and entire societies. Its prevalence shows a concerning upward trend, driven by a combination of factors such as an aging demographic, rising rates of conditions like diabetes and hypertension, and various other contributing elements. In this extensive exploration, we delve deeply into the epidemiological landscape of CKD, meticulously examining its occurrence across diverse populations and geographical regions. Through this analysis, we shed light on the substantial burden CKD imposes on healthcare systems and economies worldwide, underscoring the urgent need for comprehensive strategies to address this pressing public health issue. By comprehensively understanding the prevalence and far-reaching consequences of CKD, we gain valuable insights into the critical importance of proactive management and preventive measures. It is through this concerted effort that we can effectively mitigate the impact of CKD and safeguard the health and well-being of individuals and communities globally.

As we progress through subsequent chapters, we will traverse a plethora of topics, spanning from the anatomy and functionality of the kidneys to the various stages of CKD, diagnostic methodologies, treatment alternatives, and strategies for leading a fulfilling life with the condition. Through a comprehensive and holistic approach, our aim is to furnish readers with the knowledge, tools, and resources necessary to adeptly navigate the obstacles posed by CKD and enhance their health and well-being.

Join us as we embark on this voyage of understanding, empowerment, and optimism, equipping individuals and communities to confront CKD with resilience, determination, and hope for a brighter future.

2: ANATOMY AND FUNCTION OF THE KIDNEYS

In this expansive chapter, we embark on an enlightening exploration of the kidneys, recognizing their remarkable significance in sustaining the body's delicate balance. Through a comprehensive examination, we aim to unravel the intricacies of the kidney's intricate structure and essential functions, illuminating their role as vital organs crucial for optimal health and well-being. By delving into the anatomy of these bean-shaped marvels and elucidating their multifaceted functions, we endeavor to foster a profound appreciation for their critical importance in maintaining physiological equilibrium. Through this meticulous exploration, readers will gain a comprehensive understanding of the kidneys' intricate workings, paving the way for enhanced awareness and appreciation of their indispensable role in supporting overall health and vitality.

Structure of the Kidneys

Situated in the retroperitoneal space, on either side of the spine below the rib cage, the kidneys are paired organs. Each kidney, about the size of a fist, comprises several distinct regions:

- **Renal Cortex:** Situated at the periphery of the kidney lies the renal cortex, a region teeming with an extensive network of nephrons, the kidney's microscopic filtering units. These nephrons, numbering in the millions, serve as indispensable components in the intricate process of waste filtration and urine production. Within the renal cortex, these tiny structures meticulously extract waste products and surplus substances from the bloodstream, initiating the complex cascade of physiological events necessary for the formation of urine. Through their intricate mechanisms, the nephrons uphold the delicate balance of bodily fluids, ensuring the elimination of toxins and the maintenance of optimal physiological function. This intricate interplay underscores the pivotal role of the renal cortex and its resident nephrons in safeguarding the body's homeostasis and overall well-being.

- **Renal Medulla:** Situated beneath the renal cortex, the renal medulla comprises distinct structures known as renal pyramids, which serve as integral components of the kidney's intricate architecture. Within each pyramid, a multitude of collecting ducts can be found, tasked with the essential function of conveying urine from the nephrons to the renal pelvis. These intricate ductal networks intricately weave throughout the renal medulla, facilitating the seamless transportation of urine as it undergoes various stages of concentration and refinement. By traversing through the renal pyramids and into the renal pelvis, urine is ultimately directed towards the ureter for elimination from the body. The intricate arrangement and coordinated function of these collecting ducts within the renal medulla underscore their vital role in the renal system's overall functionality and the maintenance of fluid and electrolyte balance.

- **Renal Pelvis:** Situated as a funnel-shaped reservoir within the kidney, the renal pelvis assumes a pivotal role in the urinary system, serving as the central hub for collecting urine amassed from the intricate network of collecting ducts coursing through the renal medulla. This anatomical structure orchestrates the seamless transition of urine, channeling it towards the ureter, where it embarks on its journey for elimination from the body.

Within the intricate framework of the nephron, the renal filtration process unfolds within networks of minuscule blood vessels known as glomeruli, where blood undergoes meticulous sieving. This intricate process entails the removal of waste products, toxins, and surplus substances from the bloodstream, while preserving essential nutrients and electrolytes vital for bodily function. The resultant filtered fluid, termed filtrate, embarks on a transformative journey through various segments of the nephron, undergoing modification and concentration en route to becoming urine, ready for excretion from the body.

As the filtrate traverses through the convoluted pathways of the nephron, each segment meticulously fine-tunes its composition through processes of reabsorption, secretion, and selective permeability, orchestrated to maintain the delicate balance of bodily fluids and electrolytes. This intricate orchestration within the nephron underscores its pivotal role as the primary functional unit of the kidney, orchestrating the intricate processes essential for maintaining systemic homeostasis and overall well-being.

Functions and Importance

The kidneys perform numerous essential functions critical for maintaining overall health and well-being:

- **Filtration:** At the forefront of renal physiology lies the kidneys' paramount task of meticulously sieving waste products, toxins, and surplus substances from the circulating bloodstream, while concurrently safeguarding and preserving essential nutrients and electrolytes critical for bodily function. This intricate filtration mechanism serves as the cornerstone of renal function, orchestrating the delicate balance of bodily fluids and electrolytes to uphold systemic homeostasis and ensure optimal physiological function. By regulating the composition and volume of body fluids, the kidneys play a pivotal role in fine-tuning electrolyte concentrations and blood pressure levels, thereby safeguarding overall health and well-being. Through their multifaceted filtration processes, the kidneys emerge as indispensable guardians of systemic equilibrium, tirelessly working to maintain the delicate balance essential for sustaining vital bodily functions and promoting optimal health outcomes.

- Regulation of Fluid and Electrolyte Balance: The kidneys assume a pivotal responsibility in meticulously overseeing the equilibrium of fluids and electrolytes within the body, intricately orchestrating their levels to harmonize with the intricate web of physiological processes. Through a dynamic interplay of filtration, reabsorption, and excretion, these vital organs maintain a delicate balance, ensuring that fluid and electrolyte levels remain within narrow ranges conducive to normal bodily function. In response to fluctuations in hydration status and dietary intake, the kidneys adeptly modulate the excretion of water and electrolytes, fine-tuning their output to align with the body's evolving needs. This intricate regulatory mechanism serves as a cornerstone of renal physiology, safeguarding the body's internal milieu and preserving optimal conditions for cellular function and metabolic processes. By vigilantly monitoring and adjusting the composition of bodily fluids, the kidneys emerge as steadfast guardians of homeostasis, perpetually striving to uphold the delicate balance essential for sustaining overall health and vitality.

- **Acid-Base Balance:** A crucial aspect of renal function involves the kidneys' intricate role in managing the body's acid-base equilibrium, a vital process that ensures the pH of bodily fluids remains finely tuned within a tightly regulated range. This intricate mechanism hinges on the kidneys' ability to selectively excrete hydrogen ions while concurrently reabsorbing bicarbonate ions, thereby orchestrating the delicate balance necessary for maintaining physiological stability and optimal cellular function. Through this dynamic interplay, the kidneys serve as pivotal regulators, fine-tuning the acidity or alkalinity of bodily fluids to align with the intricate requirements of cellular metabolism and systemic homeostasis. By steadfastly navigating the flux of hydrogen and bicarbonate ions, the kidneys safeguard the body's internal environment, perpetuating an environment conducive to proper cellular function and overall physiological well-being.

- **Blood Pressure Regulation:** The kidneys play a pivotal role in regulating blood pressure through the secretion of hormones such as renin, which orchestrates the delicate balance of blood volume and systemic vascular resistance. Through this intricate hormonal regulation, the kidneys exert control over fluid retention and vascular tone, thereby contributing significantly to the maintenance of blood pressure within optimal ranges.

A profound comprehension of the intricate anatomy and indispensable functions of the kidneys is imperative, as any disruptions in renal function can precipitate a myriad of health complications. In forthcoming sections, we will embark on a comprehensive exploration of the underlying mechanisms governing kidney function, delving deeply into the intricate processes by which the kidneys filter blood, meticulously regulate fluid and electrolyte balance, and play a pivotal role in preserving the body's acid-base equilibrium.

By immersing ourselves in a detailed examination of kidney anatomy and function, readers will gain invaluable insights that will enhance their understanding of the complexities inherent in Chronic Kidney Disease. Armed with this comprehensive understanding, individuals will be better equipped to navigate the nuances of CKD, including its diagnosis, treatment modalities, and ongoing management strategies, thereby empowering them to make informed decisions regarding their health and well-being.

3: DIAGNOSING CHRONIC KIDNEY DISEASE

Within the realm of managing Chronic Kidney Disease (CKD), a critical milestone lies in the accurate diagnosis of this condition, serving as a cornerstone in preventing its progression to more advanced stages. In this chapter, we embark on a comprehensive exploration of the diverse array of screening tests, diagnostic methodologies, and procedures employed in the identification of CKD. Through meticulous examination, we delve deeply into the intricacies of these diagnostic tools, elucidating their respective roles and nuances in detecting and assessing the presence and severity of CKD.

Moreover, our exploration extends beyond the mere identification of CKD, as we underscore the paramount importance of interpreting test findings with precision and discernment. By delving into the underlying causes and contributing factors that underpin the development and progression of

CKD, we aim to shed light on the complexities inherent in its diagnosis and management. Through this comprehensive analysis, readers will gain a profound understanding of the multifaceted nature of CKD diagnosis, empowering them with the knowledge and insight necessary to navigate the diagnostic process effectively and initiate timely interventions to mitigate the impact of this chronic condition.

Screening Tests and Diagnostic Procedures

In the comprehensive screening process for Chronic Kidney Disease (CKD), a multifaceted approach is typically employed, incorporating various components such as thorough medical history assessment, comprehensive physical examination, and extensive laboratory evaluations. One of the primary screening methods frequently utilized is the measurement of serum creatinine levels, a vital parameter used to assess kidney function. This assessment is often facilitated through the application of sophisticated formulas such as the Modification of Diet in Renal Disease (MDRD) or Chronic Kidney Disease

Epidemiology Collaboration (CKD-EPI) equation, which offer valuable insights into the filtration rate of the kidneys.

Elevated serum creatinine levels serve as a notable indicator of potential compromise in kidney function, prompting the need for further diagnostic exploration and assessment. By meticulously analyzing the results of serum creatinine measurements in conjunction with other screening parameters, healthcare professionals can glean valuable information regarding the health status of the kidneys and potential indicators of CKD development. This comprehensive screening process underscores the importance of a holistic approach to CKD detection, enabling timely intervention and management strategies to mitigate the progression and impact of this chronic condition.

Moreover, urine analysis constitutes a crucial component in the comprehensive evaluation of Chronic Kidney Disease (CKD). Through meticulous examination of urine's physical and chemical properties, urinalysis serves as a valuable diagnostic tool, facilitating the detection of various abnormalities indicative of kidney dysfunction. These abnormalities may include proteinuria, hematuria, and urinary sediment, which serve as significant indicators of impaired renal function.

In addition to qualitative assessments, quantitative measures such as the urine protein-to-creatinine ratio (UPCR) and urine albumin-to-creatinine ratio (UACR) offer valuable insights into the extent of proteinuria, thereby aiding in the evaluation of kidney function. By quantifying the levels of protein excretion in relation to creatinine concentration in the urine, these measures provide clinicians with valuable data regarding the severity of kidney involvement and the progression of CKD.

The integration of urine tests into the diagnostic framework of CKD underscores the holistic approach necessary for a comprehensive evaluation of renal health. By leveraging the insights gleaned from urinalysis and quantitative assessments, healthcare providers can garner a deeper understanding of kidney function and tailor treatment strategies accordingly, thereby enhancing patient outcomes and mitigating the progression of CKD.

Additionally, imaging modalities such as ultrasound are routinely employed in the diagnostic evaluation of Chronic Kidney Disease (CKD), serving as invaluable tools for assessing various aspects of renal anatomy and structure. Through comprehensive imaging, healthcare professionals gain insights into parameters such as kidney size, shape, and structural integrity, enabling the identification of potential anatomical irregularities that may underlie or exacerbate CKD.

The utilization of ultrasound allows for meticulous scrutiny of the kidneys, facilitating the detection of abnormalities such as cysts or tumors that could impede renal function or contribute to the progression of CKD. By providing detailed visualization of renal morphology, ultrasound imaging aids in the early identification and characterization of structural anomalies, thereby facilitating timely intervention and management strategies aimed at mitigating the impact of these factors on kidney health.

The integration of imaging studies into the diagnostic armamentarium for CKD underscores the multifaceted approach required for comprehensive renal evaluation. By incorporating ultrasound assessments into the diagnostic framework, healthcare providers can glean valuable insights into renal anatomy and identify potential contributors to CKD progression, thereby optimizing patient care and outcomes through targeted interventions and therapeutic strategies.

Interpreting Test Results

Achieving a thorough understanding of test results entails a deep comprehension of the intricacies of normal kidney function and the metrics utilized to evaluate renal health. In addition to analyzing serum creatinine levels and urine tests, healthcare professionals also scrutinize a range of laboratory markers to assess kidney function and overall well-being.

These laboratory parameters encompass an array of indicators, including the estimated glomerular filtration rate (eGFR), blood urea nitrogen (BUN), and electrolyte levels. Each of these metrics offers unique insights into various aspects of renal function and health. For instance, eGFR provides an estimation of the kidneys' filtration capacity, offering valuable information regarding overall kidney function. Meanwhile, BUN levels reflect the body's urea nitrogen concentration, serving as an indicator of renal clearance and metabolic processes. Additionally, electrolyte levels offer insights into the body's fluid balance and renal electrolyte handling, further informing clinicians about kidney function and overall physiological status.

By meticulously analyzing these laboratory markers in conjunction with other diagnostic findings, healthcare providers can gain a comprehensive understanding of renal health and identify potential abnormalities or impairments in kidney function. This holistic approach to interpreting test results enables clinicians to formulate tailored treatment plans and interventions aimed at optimizing kidney health and mitigating the progression of renal disease.

The diagnosis of Chronic Kidney Disease (CKD) hinges on the persistent observation of an estimated glomerular filtration rate (eGFR) consistently below 60 mL/min/1.73 m² for a duration spanning three months or longer. This criterion serves as a pivotal threshold for identifying individuals with impaired renal function, indicating the presence of CKD. Moreover, the severity of CKD is delineated into distinct stages, with categorization based on the eGFR value and the concurrent presence of kidney damage.

A comprehensive understanding of these CKD stages is paramount, as it serves as a cornerstone for informed decision-making regarding treatment modalities and ongoing monitoring of disease progression. By familiarizing healthcare providers with the nuances of each CKD stage, clinicians can tailor treatment approaches to address specific patient needs and mitigate the risks associated with disease advancement.

Furthermore, the classification of CKD stages facilitates the establishment of personalized care plans, enabling healthcare teams to implement targeted interventions aimed at preserving kidney function and optimizing patient outcomes. Through regular monitoring and assessment of eGFR values and kidney damage indicators, clinicians can track disease progression over time, adjusting treatment strategies as necessary to effectively manage CKD and mitigate the risk of complications. This comprehensive approach underscores the importance of integrating CKD staging into clinical practice, thereby empowering healthcare providers to deliver optimal care and support to individuals living with this chronic condition.

Identifying Underlying Causes

While Chronic Kidney Disease (CKD) can arise from a multitude of factors ranging from diabetes and hypertension to autoimmune disorders, identifying the underlying cause is essential for guiding tailored treatment and management strategies. Conducting a comprehensive medical history evaluation is instrumental in unraveling the intricate web of factors contributing to CKD onset and progression. This entails delving into various facets such as familial medical history, medication usage patterns, and lifestyle factors, each of which may offer valuable insights into the root cause of CKD.

By meticulously exploring these elements, healthcare providers can gain a deeper understanding of the complex interplay of genetic predispositions, environmental influences, and lifestyle choices that may contribute to CKD development. Moreover, this holistic approach enables clinicians to discern potential risk factors and triggers associated with CKD onset, paving the way for personalized interventions aimed at addressing underlying causes and mitigating disease progression.

Furthermore, the identification of specific contributing factors through a thorough medical history assessment empowers healthcare teams to tailor treatment approaches to individual patient needs, thereby optimizing therapeutic outcomes and enhancing quality of life. Through ongoing monitoring and evaluation, clinicians can refine treatment strategies over time, ensuring that interventions remain aligned with patients' evolving needs and circumstances. This comprehensive approach underscores the importance of a multidimensional assessment in elucidating the root cause of CKD and guiding targeted interventions to mitigate its impact on patient health and well-being.

Additional diagnostic investigations may be necessary to uncover the precise underlying etiology of Chronic Kidney Disease (CKD). For example, in cases where diabetes is suspected as a contributing factor, specific blood tests assessing glucose levels and hemoglobin A1c play a pivotal role in diagnosing diabetes-related kidney disease. Similarly, comprehensive blood pressure evaluations and echocardiography examinations serve as indispensable tools for evaluating cardiovascular health and its potential impact on kidney function.

The integration of these diagnostic modalities into the evaluation process enables healthcare providers to gain deeper insights into the intricate mechanisms underlying CKD development and progression. By conducting targeted assessments tailored to individual patient needs, clinicians can identify specific risk factors and contributory elements that may be driving CKD onset or exacerbation.

Furthermore, these diagnostic tests afford clinicians the opportunity to adopt a multidimensional approach to CKD management, addressing not only the renal manifestations of the disease but also its systemic implications. Through meticulous interpretation of test results and correlation with clinical findings, healthcare teams can formulate tailored treatment plans aimed at targeting underlying causes and mitigating disease progression.

Moreover, ongoing monitoring and reassessment through serial diagnostic testing enable clinicians to track changes in disease status over time, refining treatment strategies as necessary to optimize patient outcomes and enhance long-term prognosis. This comprehensive diagnostic approach underscores the importance of a multifaceted evaluation in unraveling the complexities of CKD and guiding personalized interventions to address its underlying causes and associated comorbidities.

In specific scenarios, the consideration of a kidney biopsy may arise as a necessary step in assessing the severity of kidney damage and unraveling the underlying pathology driving Chronic Kidney Disease (CKD). This diagnostic procedure involves the extraction of a minute sample of kidney tissue for microscopic analysis, offering invaluable insights into the structural and cellular changes occurring within the kidneys.

By subjecting the biopsy specimen to detailed microscopic examination, healthcare providers gain critical diagnostic information essential for informing treatment decisions and guiding management strategies. The microscopic evaluation enables clinicians to visualize and characterize various pathological changes, such as inflammation, fibrosis, or deposition of abnormal proteins, which may be indicative of specific underlying causes or disease processes contributing to CKD.

Moreover, the insights gleaned from kidney biopsy findings facilitate the formulation of personalized treatment approaches tailored to address the specific pathological mechanisms driving CKD in each individual case. This targeted therapeutic approach aims to mitigate disease progression, alleviate symptoms, and preserve kidney function to the greatest extent possible.

However, it is important to recognize that kidney biopsy is not without risks, and its utilization must be carefully weighed against potential benefits and patient-specific factors. Therefore, the decision to proceed with a kidney biopsy should be made in close collaboration between healthcare providers and patients, taking into consideration the overall clinical context and individual circumstances.

Kidney biopsy represents a valuable diagnostic tool in the comprehensive evaluation of CKD, offering unique insights into the underlying pathology and guiding personalized treatment strategies aimed at optimizing patient outcomes. Through judicious utilization and meticulous interpretation of biopsy findings, healthcare providers can effectively tailor interventions to address the specific pathological processes driving CKD progression, thereby enhancing the quality of care and improving long-term prognosis.

In summary, the diagnosis of Chronic Kidney Disease (CKD) necessitates a comprehensive and multidimensional approach that encompasses a variety of screening tests, thorough interpretation of test results, and identification of underlying contributing factors. By integrating diverse diagnostic methodologies and tools, healthcare practitioners can effectively diagnose CKD, thereby initiating appropriate treatment interventions and implementing personalized management strategies tailored to each patient's unique needs. Early detection and intervention play a crucial role in slowing disease progression and preserving kidney function, ultimately leading to improved quality of life for individuals affected by CKD.

To achieve an accurate diagnosis of CKD, healthcare professionals must employ a multifaceted diagnostic strategy that includes screening tests to detect early signs of renal dysfunction, meticulous interpretation of test findings to identify specific markers indicative of CKD, and an in-depth investigation into potential underlying causes such as diabetes, hypertension, or autoimmune disorders. By conducting a thorough assessment and considering all relevant clinical factors, clinicians can establish a precise diagnosis of CKD and initiate appropriate treatment measures promptly.

Furthermore, the implementation of tailored management strategies is essential in optimizing patient outcomes and mitigating the impact of CKD on overall health and well-being. This may involve a combination of lifestyle modifications, pharmacological interventions, and therapeutic approaches aimed at slowing disease progression, managing symptoms, and preventing complications. By addressing CKD comprehensively and proactively, healthcare providers can improve patient outcomes and enhance quality of life for individuals living with this chronic condition.

In essence, the diagnosis of CKD is a complex process that requires a holistic and individualized approach. Through careful consideration of screening results, thorough interpretation of diagnostic tests, and targeted investigation into underlying causes, healthcare practitioners can effectively diagnose CKD, initiate appropriate treatment interventions, and implement tailored management strategies to optimize patient outcomes and improve quality of life.

4: STAGES OF CHRONIC KIDNEY DISEASE

Understanding the various stages of Chronic Kidney Disease (CKD) is essential for devising effective management strategies and predicting patient outcomes. In this chapter, we embark on an in-depth exploration of the CKD stages, delving into the nuanced progression of the disease and emphasizing the importance of ongoing monitoring to optimize patient care and prognosis.

Through comprehensive analysis and examination, we aim to provide a comprehensive overview of the stages of CKD, elucidating the distinct characteristics and clinical implications associated with each stage. By scrutinizing the evolving nature of CKD progression, healthcare practitioners can gain valuable insights into the trajectory of the disease and tailor treatment approaches accordingly.
Furthermore, we underscore the significance of continuous monitoring in the management of

CKD, emphasizing the need for regular assessments to track disease progression, monitor treatment efficacy, and identify potential complications. By adopting a proactive approach to patient care, healthcare providers can intervene early to mitigate the impact of CKD and optimize patient outcomes.

Through an exploration of the CKD stages and the imperative of continual monitoring, we aim to equip healthcare professionals with the knowledge and tools necessary to effectively manage this chronic condition. By fostering a deeper understanding of CKD progression and the importance of vigilant monitoring, we empower healthcare practitioners to deliver personalized and comprehensive care that enhances patient well-being and quality of life.

Overview of CKD Stages:

Chronic Kidney Disease is classified into five stages based on the severity of kidney damage and the level of kidney function, as assessed by the estimated glomerular filtration rate (eGFR). These stages are outlined as follows:

Stage 1: In the initial stage of Chronic Kidney Disease (CKD), known as Stage 1, patients exhibit kidney damage alongside either normal or increased estimated glomerular filtration rate (eGFR), which typically exceeds 90 mL/min/1.73 m². While signs of kidney damage, such as proteinuria or abnormal imaging findings, may manifest, kidney function remains relatively intact during this early phase.

Within Stage 1 CKD, individuals may experience subtle indicators of renal impairment, including the presence of proteinuria or abnormalities detected through imaging studies. Despite these early signs of kidney damage, patients typically maintain adequate kidney function, as evidenced by the eGFR exceeding the normal threshold.

This stage serves as a critical juncture in the progression of CKD, as it offers an opportunity for early detection and intervention to mitigate further kidney damage and slow disease progression. By identifying and addressing underlying risk factors and implementing targeted interventions, healthcare providers can potentially delay or prevent the onset of more advanced stages of

CKD, thereby optimizing patient outcomes and quality of life.

Through vigilant monitoring and proactive management strategies, individuals diagnosed with Stage 1 CKD can be afforded the opportunity to enact lifestyle modifications, adhere to treatment regimens, and engage in preventative measures aimed at preserving kidney function and mitigating the impact of the disease on overall health and well-being.

Stage 2: In Stage 2 of Chronic Kidney Disease (CKD), patients typically experience a mild decline in estimated glomerular filtration rate (eGFR), ranging from 60 to 89 mL/min/1.73 m². At this stage, evidence of kidney damage persists, accompanied by a slight impairment in kidney function. However, individuals may not exhibit overt symptoms or manifestations of renal dysfunction during this phase.

During Stage 2 CKD, patients may undergo subtle changes in renal function, as reflected by the gradual decline in eGFR. Despite this mild reduction in kidney function, the impairment remains relatively modest, and individuals may not perceive any noticeable symptoms or adverse effects on their daily activities.

Although kidney damage persists from the preceding stage, the clinical presentation of Stage 2 CKD may not be readily apparent, underscoring the importance of vigilant monitoring and proactive management strategies. Healthcare providers must remain vigilant in detecting early signs of renal impairment and implementing interventions aimed at slowing disease progression and preserving kidney function.

Through targeted interventions such as lifestyle modifications, medication management, and close monitoring of renal parameters, individuals diagnosed with Stage 2 CKD can potentially delay the onset of more advanced stages of the disease and maintain optimal health outcomes. This stage serves as a critical opportunity for early intervention and proactive management, emphasizing the importance of comprehensive care and regular follow-up appointments to optimize patient well-being and quality of life.

Stage 3: In Stage 3 of Chronic Kidney Disease (CKD), patients demonstrate a moderate decline in estimated glomerular filtration rate (eGFR), typically ranging from 30 to 59 mL/min/1.73 m². This stage is further subdivided into Stage 3a, characterized by an eGFR of 45 to 59 mL/min/1.73 m², and Stage 3b, marked by an eGFR of 30 to 44 mL/min/1.73 m². At this juncture, individuals may begin to experience noticeable symptoms and complications associated with CKD.

During Stage 3 CKD, the decline in eGFR indicates a progressive deterioration in kidney function, albeit at a moderate pace. This reduction in kidney function is accompanied by a heightened risk of developing complications and experiencing symptomatic manifestations of renal dysfunction.

The subdivision of Stage 3 CKD into Stage 3a and Stage 3b allows for a more nuanced assessment of disease severity and helps guide treatment decisions and management strategies. Individuals in Stage 3a may exhibit milder symptoms and complications compared to those in Stage 3b, where the decline in eGFR approaches the lower end of the spectrum.
Symptoms and complications associated with Stage 3 CKD may include fatigue, fluid retention, electrolyte imbalances, and anemia, among others. These manifestations underscore the importance of proactive management and timely interventions to

mitigate the impact of CKD on overall health and well-being.

Through close monitoring, symptom management, and implementation of targeted interventions such as medication adjustments and lifestyle modifications, healthcare providers can optimize patient outcomes and enhance quality of life for individuals navigating Stage 3 CKD. This stage represents a critical juncture in the disease trajectory, emphasizing the importance of comprehensive care and multidisciplinary support to address the evolving needs of patients with CKD.

Stage 4: In Stage 4 of Chronic Kidney Disease (CKD), individuals exhibit a pronounced decline in estimated glomerular filtration rate (eGFR), typically falling within the range of 15 to 29 mL/min/1.73 m². At this advanced stage, patients face an elevated risk of developing complications such as anemia, bone disease, and cardiovascular issues, stemming from the significant impairment in kidney function.

The profound reduction in eGFR observed in Stage 4 CKD underscores the severity of renal dysfunction experienced by affected individuals. This substantial decline in kidney function significantly compromises the body's ability to effectively filter waste products and maintain fluid and electrolyte balance, predisposing patients to a myriad of complications and adverse health outcomes.

Complications commonly associated with Stage 4 CKD include anemia, resulting from decreased production of erythropoietin by the kidneys, as well as bone disease characterized by abnormalities in bone metabolism and mineralization. Additionally, individuals in this stage are at heightened risk of developing cardiovascular issues such as hypertension, heart failure, and coronary artery disease, due to the interplay between impaired kidney function and cardiovascular health.

The management of Stage 4 CKD necessitates a comprehensive and multidisciplinary approach aimed at addressing both the underlying renal dysfunction and associated complications. Treatment strategies may include pharmacological interventions to manage symptoms and complications, dietary modifications to mitigate the progression of kidney disease, and lifestyle changes to optimize cardiovascular health and overall well-being.

Furthermore, close monitoring of renal function, symptom management, and regular follow-up appointments are essential components of Stage 4 CKD management, enabling healthcare providers to assess disease progression, adjust treatment regimens, and provide timely interventions to mitigate the impact of CKD on patient health and quality of life.

In conclusion, Stage 4 CKD represents a critical juncture in the disease trajectory, characterized by a significant decline in kidney function and a heightened risk of complications. Through comprehensive care and proactive management, healthcare providers can optimize patient outcomes and enhance quality of life for individuals navigating this advanced stage of CKD.

Stage 5: At the final stage of Chronic Kidney Disease (CKD), denoted by an estimated glomerular filtration rate (eGFR) of less than 15 mL/min/1.73 m², individuals reach a critical juncture characterized by kidney failure or end-stage renal disease (ESRD). In this advanced stage, renal function is severely compromised, posing significant challenges to the body's ability to effectively filter waste products and maintain fluid and electrolyte balance.

Individuals in this stage of CKD face a profound decline in kidney function, necessitating prompt intervention to sustain life and preserve overall health. With an eGFR below 15 mL/min/1.73 m², patients are at imminent risk of experiencing life-threatening complications and adverse health outcomes.

Given the severity of renal dysfunction observed in kidney failure or ESRD, renal replacement therapy becomes imperative to sustain vital physiological functions and maintain quality of life. Options for renal replacement therapy include dialysis, which involves the artificial filtration of blood to remove waste products and excess fluids, or kidney transplantation, where a healthy kidney from a donor is surgically implanted to replace the non-functioning kidneys.

The decision to initiate renal replacement therapy is guided by various factors, including the individual's overall health status, presence of comorbidities, personal preferences, and availability of resources. Healthcare providers work closely with patients to explore the most suitable treatment option based on their unique circumstances and goals of care.

In addition to renal replacement therapy, individuals with kidney failure or ESRD require comprehensive medical management to address associated complications and optimize overall health outcomes. This may include pharmacological interventions to manage symptoms, dietary modifications to maintain nutritional balance, and close monitoring to assess treatment efficacy and disease progression.

In conclusion, kidney failure or end-stage renal disease represents the most advanced stage of CKD, characterized by severely compromised renal function and a heightened risk of complications. Through timely intervention and comprehensive management, healthcare providers strive to optimize patient outcomes and enhance quality of life for individuals navigating this critical phase of kidney disease.

Progression and Monitoring

The advancement of Chronic Kidney Disease (CKD) through its various stages can vary significantly among individuals and is influenced by a multitude of factors, including the underlying cause of kidney disease, concurrent health conditions, and lifestyle choices. While some patients may experience a rapid deterioration in kidney function, others may undergo a more gradual progression over time.

It is essential to recognize that the trajectory of CKD progression is not uniform and can vary greatly from person to person. Factors such as genetic predisposition, comorbidities like diabetes or hypertension, and lifestyle habits such as diet and exercise can all impact the rate at which CKD advances.

Given the variability in CKD progression, continuous monitoring of kidney function and disease advancement is paramount in managing the condition and mitigating associated complications. Healthcare providers conduct regular assessments of key parameters such as estimated glomerular filtration rate (eGFR), urine protein levels, blood pressure, and electrolyte balance to monitor changes in renal function and identify signs of disease progression or complications.

These ongoing evaluations enable healthcare teams to tailor treatment strategies and interventions to each individual's unique needs, optimizing outcomes and enhancing quality of life. By closely monitoring CKD progression and adjusting management plans accordingly, healthcare providers can help slow the advancement of the disease, minimize complications, and improve overall patient outcomes.

Furthermore, patient education and empowerment play a crucial role in CKD management, as individuals are encouraged to actively participate in their care by adhering to prescribed treatments, making lifestyle modifications, and attending regular follow-up appointments. Through collaborative efforts between patients and healthcare providers, the impact of CKD can be effectively managed, promoting better health outcomes and quality of life for those affected by this chronic condition.

Treatment strategies are customized to correspond with each stage of Chronic Kidney Disease (CKD), prioritizing the objectives of slowing disease progression, alleviating symptoms, and managing concurrent complications. A holistic approach is adopted, integrating lifestyle modifications and pharmacological interventions tailored to the individual's unique needs and health status.

In alignment with the stage-specific management approach, lifestyle adjustments constitute a cornerstone of CKD treatment. Encouraging dietary modifications, weight management strategies, and smoking cessation initiatives are pivotal components aimed at optimizing overall health and mitigating risk factors associated with CKD progression. These lifestyle modifications are complemented by pharmacological interventions targeted at controlling blood pressure, managing cholesterol levels, and addressing other comorbidities that may coexist with CKD.
As CKD advances to more severe stages, the consideration of renal replacement therapy

becomes imperative to sustain vital bodily functions and improve quality of life. Options such as hemodialysis, peritoneal dialysis, and kidney transplantation are evaluated, with the choice of treatment modality guided by individual factors such as age, overall health status, and personal preferences.

Central to effective CKD management is the establishment of regular follow-up appointments with healthcare providers, encompassing nephrologists and primary care physicians. These ongoing evaluations serve as opportunities for monitoring CKD progression, assessing treatment efficacy, and addressing any emerging concerns or complications. Through collaborative discussions and shared decision-making, healthcare teams and patients work together to optimize treatment plans and enhance overall outcomes.

Patient education and empowerment are integral components of CKD management, fostering active engagement in self-care practices, medication adherence, and lifestyle adjustments. By equipping individuals with the knowledge and tools necessary to navigate their condition, patient empowerment facilitates informed decision-making and promotes a sense of autonomy and control over one's health journey.

CKD management encompasses a multifaceted and individualized approach, incorporating lifestyle modifications, pharmacological interventions, and renal replacement therapy as necessary. Regular monitoring and patient education serve as pillars of effective CKD care, promoting optimal outcomes and quality of life for individuals affected by this chronic condition.
In conclusion, comprehending the stages of Chronic Kidney Disease is pivotal for guiding treatment decisions, tracking disease progression, and enhancing patient outcomes. By recognizing the distinct stages and implementing appropriate management strategies, healthcare professionals can effectively delay disease advancement, alleviate symptoms, and enhance the quality of life for individuals grappling with CKD. Consistent monitoring and proactive management are pivotal in ensuring optimal outcomes for patients across all stages of the condition.

5: TREATMENT OPTIONS FOR CHRONIC KIDNEY DISEASE

Managing Chronic Kidney Disease (CKD) effectively requires a multifaceted strategy encompassing medications, lifestyle adjustments, and dietary changes. This chapter explores the diverse treatment avenues available for CKD, focusing on medications for symptom control, lifestyle modifications to foster kidney health, and dietary adjustments tailored to individual needs.

Medications for Symptom Management

Though CKD lacks a cure, medications are pivotal in symptom alleviation and disease progression retardation. Various medication classes are prescribed for CKD to target specific symptoms and complications:

1. Blood Pressure Medications: Addressing hypertension plays a crucial role in the management of Chronic Kidney Disease (CKD), as it can exacerbate renal damage and accelerate disease progression. To effectively manage blood pressure in CKD patients, healthcare providers commonly prescribe medications such as Angiotensin-Converting Enzyme (ACE) inhibitors and Angiotensin II Receptor Blockers (ARBs). These medications are recommended for their ability to regulate blood pressure and provide renal protection by mitigating further harm to the kidneys.

The management of hypertension in CKD involves a comprehensive approach that aims to achieve optimal blood pressure control while minimizing adverse effects and preserving kidney function. In addition to pharmacological interventions, lifestyle modifications such as dietary changes, weight management, and regular exercise are encouraged to further support blood pressure management and overall cardiovascular health.

ACE inhibitors and ARBs are particularly favored in CKD management due to their specific mechanisms of action, which target the renin-angiotensin-aldosterone system (RAAS) to regulate blood pressure and reduce renal inflammation and fibrosis. By blocking the actions of angiotensin II, these medications help dilate blood vessels, decrease fluid retention, and improve renal blood flow, thereby protecting the kidneys from further damage.

Furthermore, the use of ACE inhibitors and ARBs in CKD management extends beyond blood pressure control, as they have been shown to exert renoprotective effects independent of their antihypertensive properties. These medications may help slow the progression of CKD, delay the need for renal replacement therapy, and improve long-term outcomes for patients with renal dysfunction.

However, it is important to recognize that the use of ACE inhibitors and ARBs in CKD management requires careful monitoring and individualized treatment adjustments based on patient response, renal function, and the presence of comorbidities. Close collaboration between healthcare providers and patients is essential to optimize blood pressure management and renal protection while minimizing potential adverse effects associated with these medications.

In summary, the use of ACE inhibitors and ARBs represents a cornerstone of hypertension management in CKD, offering both blood pressure control and renoprotective benefits. These medications, when used in conjunction with lifestyle modifications and regular monitoring, play a pivotal role in preserving kidney function and improving outcomes for individuals with CKD.

2. Anemia Medications: Anemia is a prevalent complication in Chronic Kidney Disease (CKD), primarily attributed to diminished erythropoietin production by the kidneys. To effectively manage anemia in CKD patients, healthcare providers often prescribe Erythropoiesis-Stimulating Agents (ESAs) such as erythropoietin and darbepoetin. These medications are utilized to stimulate the production of red blood cells, thereby alleviating symptoms associated with anemia and improving overall quality of life for affected individuals.

The management of anemia in CKD necessitates a multifaceted approach that addresses both the underlying cause of reduced erythropoietin production and the associated symptoms of anemia. ESAs serve as a cornerstone of treatment by augmenting the body's natural production of red blood cells, thereby increasing hemoglobin levels and improving oxygen delivery to tissues throughout the body.

The use of ESAs in CKD management is supported by their ability to mimic the action of endogenous erythropoietin, stimulating erythropoiesis and promoting the maturation and proliferation of red blood cell precursors in the bone marrow. By enhancing red blood cell production, ESAs help alleviate symptoms of anemia such as fatigue, weakness, and shortness of breath, thereby enhancing quality of life and functional status in CKD patients.

Furthermore, ESAs are administered through various routes, including subcutaneous injection or intravenous infusion, with dosing regimens tailored to individual patient characteristics and treatment goals. Close monitoring of hemoglobin levels and iron status is essential to optimize ESA therapy and minimize the risk of adverse effects such as hypertension, thrombosis, and pure red cell aplasia.

In addition to ESA therapy, the management of anemia in CKD may involve other interventions such as iron supplementation, erythropoietin-stimulating agents, and blood transfusions, depending on the severity of anemia and the presence of underlying comorbidities. Healthcare providers work collaboratively with patients to develop individualized treatment plans that address their unique needs and preferences while maximizing therapeutic efficacy and minimizing risks.

In summary, the use of Erythropoiesis-Stimulating Agents represents a key component of anemia management in CKD, offering a targeted approach to stimulating red blood cell production and alleviating symptoms of anemia. Through careful monitoring and individualized treatment adjustments, healthcare providers can optimize ESA therapy to improve hemoglobin levels, enhance quality of life, and promote overall well-being in CKD patients affected by anemia.

3. Phosphate Binders: Chronic Kidney Disease (CKD) frequently results in disruptions to mineral metabolism, leading to elevated phosphate levels in the bloodstream. To address this imbalance and mitigate the risk of complications such as bone disease and cardiovascular issues, healthcare providers often prescribe phosphate binders. These medications, available in both calcium-based and non-calcium-based formulations, function by binding to dietary phosphate in the gastrointestinal tract, thereby preventing its absorption into the bloodstream.

The management of abnormal phosphate levels in CKD requires a comprehensive approach aimed at controlling phosphate absorption while preserving overall mineral balance and bone health. Phosphate binders play a central role in this strategy by effectively reducing the concentration of phosphate in the bloodstream, thereby minimizing the risk of complications associated with hyperphosphatemia.

Calcium-based phosphate binders, such as calcium carbonate or calcium acetate, work by binding to dietary phosphate in the gut and forming insoluble complexes that are subsequently excreted in the feces. These agents not only lower phosphate levels but also provide supplemental calcium, which may be beneficial for maintaining bone density and reducing the risk of osteoporosis in CKD patients.

Non-calcium-based phosphate binders, such as sevelamer or lanthanum carbonate, offer an alternative treatment option for CKD patients who are unable to tolerate or require additional phosphate control beyond what calcium-based binders can provide. These agents function by binding to phosphate in the gastrointestinal tract without contributing to calcium or aluminum load, making them suitable for patients with hypercalcemia or aluminum toxicity.

In addition to phosphate binders, dietary phosphate restriction and optimization of renal function are important components of managing hyperphosphatemia in CKD. Healthcare providers work collaboratively with patients to develop individualized treatment plans that incorporate lifestyle modifications, dietary counseling, and medication management to achieve optimal phosphate control and mitigate the risk of associated complications.

Regular monitoring of serum phosphate levels and renal function is essential to assess treatment efficacy and adjust therapy as necessary. Close communication between healthcare providers and patients facilitates shared decision-making and ensures that treatment plans are tailored to each individual's unique needs and preferences.

In summary, phosphate binders represent a cornerstone of management for hyperphosphatemia in CKD, offering an effective means of controlling phosphate levels and reducing the risk of complications such as bone disease and cardiovascular issues. Through comprehensive treatment strategies that encompass lifestyle modifications, dietary interventions, and medication management, healthcare providers strive to optimize phosphate control and improve outcomes for CKD patients affected by abnormal mineral metabolism.

4. Diuretics: Diuretics play a crucial role in the management of Chronic Kidney Disease (CKD) by helping to regulate fluid balance and alleviate symptoms associated with fluid retention, such as edema and hypertension. Among the various classes of diuretics available, loop diuretics such as furosemide and thiazide diuretics are frequently employed to augment urine output and reduce fluid overload in CKD patients.

The use of diuretics in CKD management is aimed at addressing the impaired renal function that often leads to fluid retention and volume overload. By promoting diuresis and increasing urinary excretion of sodium and water, diuretics help to alleviate symptoms of fluid overload such as peripheral edema, pulmonary congestion, and hypertension.

Loop diuretics, such as furosemide, exert their effects by inhibiting the reabsorption of sodium and chloride ions in the ascending limb of the loop of Henle, leading to increased urinary sodium and water excretion. These agents are particularly effective in managing volume overload and reducing extracellular fluid volume in CKD patients with impaired renal function.

Thiazide diuretics, on the other hand, act on the distal convoluted tubule of the nephron to inhibit sodium reabsorption, thereby promoting diuresis and reducing blood volume and systemic vascular resistance. While thiazide diuretics are less potent than loop diuretics, they may be used in combination with other diuretics or as adjunctive therapy in CKD patients with mild to moderate volume overload.

The choice of diuretic therapy in CKD management is guided by various factors, including the severity of fluid overload, renal function, electrolyte balance, and individual patient characteristics. Healthcare providers work collaboratively with patients to develop personalized treatment plans that optimize diuretic therapy while minimizing the risk of adverse effects such as electrolyte imbalances, hypotension, and renal impairment.

Regular monitoring of fluid status, renal function, and electrolyte levels is essential to assess the efficacy and safety of diuretic therapy in CKD patients. Close communication between healthcare providers and patients facilitates ongoing evaluation and adjustment of treatment regimens to achieve optimal fluid balance and symptom relief while minimizing the risk of complications.

In summary, diuretics represent an important component of CKD management, offering effective relief from symptoms of fluid overload and hypertension. Through individualized treatment strategies and close monitoring, healthcare providers strive to optimize diuretic therapy and improve outcomes for CKD patients affected by impaired fluid balance.

Lifestyle Modifications for Kidney Health

In conjunction with medications, lifestyle alterations are pivotal for fostering kidney health and impeding CKD progression. Several lifestyle changes are instrumental in enhancing CKD management:

1. Regular Exercise: Consistent physical activity improves cardiovascular health, mitigates blood pressure, and diminishes CKD-related complications risk. Strive for at least 30 minutes of moderate-intensity exercise most days of the week, as endorsed by healthcare providers.

2. Smoking Cessation: Smoking exacerbates CKD progression and negatively impacts kidney function. Ceasing smoking can decelerate CKD progression and lessen associated cardiovascular risks.

3. Weight Management: Maintaining a healthy weight is critical for CKD management and curbing risks like diabetes and hypertension. A balanced diet and regular exercise are pivotal for achieving and sustaining a healthy weight, thereby augmenting kidney function and overall health.

4. Blood Pressure Regulation: Keeping blood pressure within target ranges is pivotal for CKD patients to retard kidney damage progression. Adhering to healthcare provider recommendations for blood pressure monitoring and medication adherence is crucial for maintaining optimal blood pressure levels.

Dietary Adjustments for Kidney Disease

Dietary modifications play a pivotal role in CKD management by mitigating symptoms, averting complications, and stalling disease progression. Tailored dietary adjustments include:

1. Sodium Reduction: Limiting sodium intake is imperative in the management of Chronic Kidney Disease (CKD) as it plays a pivotal role in mitigating fluid retention and hypertension, both prevalent complications of the condition. The recommended daily target for sodium consumption is set at less than 2,300 milligrams, although a more stringent reduction may be warranted if blood pressure control remains inadequate.

Managing sodium intake is essential in CKD management due to its significant impact on fluid balance and blood pressure regulation. Excessive sodium consumption can exacerbate fluid retention and volume overload, thereby intensifying symptoms like edema while heightening the risk of hypertension and associated cardiovascular complications.

By adhering to a reduced sodium diet, individuals with CKD can alleviate stress on the kidneys and cardiovascular system, promoting overall health and enhancing quality of life. Dietary modifications aimed at sodium reduction may involve prioritizing fresh, whole foods over processed and packaged options, which are often laden with sodium. Awareness of hidden sources of sodium in condiments, sauces, and pre-packaged meals is also crucial, empowering individuals to make informed choices and minimize sodium intake effectively.

Regular monitoring of blood pressure and fluid status is pivotal for CKD patients following a sodium-restricted diet, facilitating adjustments as needed to optimize treatment outcomes. Collaborative efforts between healthcare providers and patients are instrumental in devising personalized dietary plans that align with sodium intake recommendations while accommodating individual preferences and nutritional requirements.

In summary, prioritizing sodium reduction constitutes a cornerstone of CKD management, offering multifaceted benefits in terms of fluid balance regulation and blood pressure management. Through conscious dietary adjustments and proactive lifestyle modifications, individuals with CKD can actively contribute to their overall well-being and reduce the risk of complications associated with excess sodium consumption..

2. Protein Limitation: Limiting protein intake is often a crucial consideration for individuals with advanced Chronic Kidney Disease (CKD) to alleviate the workload on the kidneys and address complications such as proteinuria and uremia. Working in tandem with a registered dietitian is recommended to determine the optimal protein intake tailored to individual factors such as kidney function and overall nutritional status.

Restricting protein consumption is a key aspect of managing advanced CKD, as it serves to lessen the burden on the kidneys and mitigate potential complications associated with impaired renal function. By reducing protein intake, individuals with CKD can help to minimize the excretion of waste products and metabolic byproducts, thereby alleviating stress on the kidneys and promoting renal health.

Collaboration with a registered dietitian is invaluable in establishing personalized dietary plans that strike a balance between adequate nutrition and renal preservation. Factors such as the stage of CKD, degree of kidney impairment, and individual dietary preferences and requirements are carefully considered to determine the appropriate level of protein restriction.

The role of protein in the diet of individuals with CKD is multifaceted, as it is essential for supporting various bodily functions while also posing challenges in terms of renal handling and metabolism. By tailoring protein intake to individual needs and circumstances, healthcare providers can optimize nutritional support while minimizing the risk of exacerbating kidney dysfunction.

Regular monitoring of kidney function and nutritional status is essential for individuals with CKD following a protein-restricted diet, allowing for adjustments as needed to optimize dietary management and overall health outcomes. Open communication and ongoing collaboration between healthcare providers and patients facilitate informed decision-making and empower individuals to take an active role in managing their condition.
In summary, protein limitation represents an important component of dietary management in

advanced CKD, offering benefits in terms of alleviating kidney workload and mitigating complications associated with impaired renal function. Through personalized dietary planning and collaborative care, individuals with CKD can optimize their nutritional intake while promoting renal health and overall well-being.

3. Potassium and Phosphorus Management:
Vigilant monitoring of potassium and phosphorus intake is essential for individuals with Chronic Kidney Disease (CKD) to prevent electrolyte imbalances and mitigate the risk of complications such as hyperkalemia and hyperphosphatemia. Managing dietary sources of these minerals is paramount, with a focus on limiting consumption of high-potassium and high-phosphorus foods and beverages to maintain optimal electrolyte levels.

The careful regulation of potassium and phosphorus intake is a critical aspect of CKD management, as disturbances in these electrolytes can have profound implications for renal function and overall health. Excessive potassium intake can lead to hyperkalemia, characterized by elevated serum potassium levels and an increased risk of cardiac arrhythmias and other cardiovascular complications. Similarly, elevated phosphorus levels can contribute to hyperphosphatemia, which is associated with vascular calcification, bone disease, and cardiovascular morbidity and mortality in CKD patients.

To mitigate the risk of electrolyte imbalances and associated complications, CKD patients are advised to adopt dietary strategies aimed at reducing potassium and phosphorus intake. This may involve limiting consumption of potassium-rich foods such as bananas, oranges, tomatoes, potatoes, and dairy products, as well as avoiding high-phosphorus foods like processed meats, cheese, nuts, and certain beverages.

Collaboration with a registered dietitian is essential to develop individualized dietary plans that strike a balance between adequate nutrition and electrolyte management. Factors such as the stage of CKD, degree of renal impairment, and presence of comorbidities are taken into account when devising dietary recommendations tailored to each patient's specific needs and circumstances.

Regular monitoring of serum potassium and phosphorus levels, as well as renal function, is integral to assessing the effectiveness of dietary interventions and making adjustments as needed to optimize electrolyte balance and overall health outcomes. Open communication and ongoing collaboration between healthcare providers and patients facilitate informed decision-making and empower individuals to take an active role in managing their condition.

In summary, potassium and phosphorus management represent fundamental aspects of dietary management in CKD, offering benefits in terms of preventing electrolyte imbalances and mitigating complications associated with impaired renal function. Through personalized dietary planning and collaborative care, individuals with CKD can optimize their nutritional intake while promoting renal health and overall well-being.

4. Fluid Regulation: Careful monitoring of fluid intake is crucial for individuals with Chronic Kidney Disease (CKD), especially those experiencing fluid retention or undergoing dialysis treatment. Adhering to the fluid intake restrictions advised by healthcare professionals is essential to manage complications such as edema, hypertension, and electrolyte imbalances effectively.

Maintaining a vigilant approach to fluid regulation is paramount for CKD patients, as excessive fluid intake can exacerbate symptoms and complications associated with impaired renal function. By closely monitoring fluid intake and adhering to prescribed limitations, individuals with CKD can help mitigate the risk of fluid overload and its adverse consequences.

The management of fluid intake in CKD involves striking a delicate balance between maintaining adequate hydration and preventing fluid retention. Healthcare professionals may recommend specific fluid intake targets based on individual factors such as kidney function, urinary output, and presence of comorbidities.

For CKD patients undergoing dialysis treatment, fluid intake restrictions are particularly important to prevent volume overload during dialysis sessions and minimize the risk of complications such as hypotension and electrolyte imbalances. Following dietary and fluid intake guidelines provided by healthcare providers is essential for optimizing the effectiveness and safety of dialysis therapy.

In addition to adhering to fluid intake restrictions, CKD patients are encouraged to adopt lifestyle modifications that promote overall fluid balance and kidney health. This may include reducing intake of high-sodium foods and beverages, engaging in regular physical activity, and managing underlying conditions such as hypertension and diabetes.

Regular monitoring of fluid status, blood pressure, and electrolyte levels is essential for assessing the effectiveness of fluid regulation strategies and making adjustments as needed to optimize patient outcomes. Collaborative communication between healthcare providers and patients fosters shared decision-making and empowers individuals to take an active role in managing their fluid intake and overall health.

In summary, vigilant monitoring and adherence to fluid intake restrictions are essential components of CKD management, offering benefits in terms of preventing complications and optimizing renal health. Through personalized guidance and ongoing support from healthcare professionals, individuals with CKD can achieve better fluid balance and improve their overall well-being.

In conclusion, treating Chronic Kidney Disease necessitates a comprehensive approach, integrating medications, lifestyle modifications, and tailored dietary adjustments. By mitigating symptoms, managing risk factors, and fostering kidney health, CKD patients can decelerate disease progression, alleviate complications, and enhance overall quality of life. Close collaboration with healthcare providers and adherence to treatment plans are pivotal for optimizing outcomes and sustaining kidney health in individuals grappling with CKD.

6: ADVANCED TREATMENT MODALITIES

As Chronic Kidney Disease (CKD) progresses to severe stages, the necessity for more intensive treatment approaches becomes paramount to ensure both survival and the maintenance of a satisfactory quality of life. This segment delves comprehensively into the advanced treatment modalities available for CKD, encompassing a range of interventions such as hemodialysis and peritoneal dialysis, kidney transplantation, and palliative care tailored specifically for individuals grappling with end-stage kidney disease.

Hemodialysis and Peritoneal Dialysis

Both hemodialysis and peritoneal dialysis serve as forms of renal replacement therapy aimed at eliminating waste products and excess fluids from the body when the kidneys can no longer adequately perform these functions.

1. Hemodialysis: Hemodialysis involves the use of a medical apparatus called a hemodialyzer, which is designed to filter blood outside the body. This process, usually administered at a specialized facility known as a dialysis center, occurs multiple times per week and can last for several hours each session.

During hemodialysis, blood is drawn from the patient's body and directed into the hemodialyzer. Within this device, the blood passes through a selectively permeable membrane, which effectively separates waste products and excess fluids from the bloodstream. These unwanted substances are then removed from the blood, leaving it purified and cleansed.

Following this purification process, the filtered blood is returned to the patient's body, where it can continue its vital functions. This intricate procedure serves a critical role in managing Chronic Kidney Disease (CKD) by aiding in the elimination of toxins and regulating fluid levels within the body.

Hemodialysis sessions are meticulously supervised by trained healthcare professionals to ensure the safety and effectiveness of the treatment. Patients undergoing hemodialysis often require regular monitoring of their vital signs and blood chemistry to optimize their treatment regimen and overall well-being. Through hemodialysis, individuals with advanced CKD can sustain their health and quality of life despite the challenges posed by their condition.

2. Peritoneal Dialysis: Peritoneal dialysis utilizes the peritoneum, a membrane that lines the abdominal cavity, as a natural filtration system. Unlike hemodialysis, which is conducted in a dialysis center, peritoneal dialysis can be performed at home, providing patients with increased flexibility and independence in managing their treatment regimen.

During peritoneal dialysis, a sterile dialysis solution is introduced into the abdominal cavity through a catheter. Once inside the peritoneum, the solution acts as a filter, absorbing waste products and excess fluids from the bloodstream. This process occurs over a period known as the dwell time, during which the solution remains in the abdomen to facilitate the exchange of fluids and solutes.

After the dwell time, the used dialysis solution, along with the waste products and excess fluids it has absorbed, is drained from the abdomen and discarded. This cycle is typically repeated multiple times throughout the day, depending on the patient's prescribed treatment regimen.

Peritoneal dialysis offers several advantages over hemodialysis, including the ability to perform the procedure at home and on a more flexible schedule. This allows patients to integrate their treatment into their daily lives more seamlessly and reduces the need for frequent visits to a dialysis center.

However, peritoneal dialysis also requires careful attention to hygiene and infection control, as the catheter insertion site must be kept clean and free from contamination to prevent complications such as peritonitis. Additionally, patients undergoing peritoneal dialysis may require ongoing monitoring and adjustments to their treatment plan to ensure optimal outcomes and minimize the risk of complications.

Overall, peritoneal dialysis represents a valuable treatment option for individuals with Chronic Kidney Disease, offering both clinical efficacy and the opportunity for enhanced quality of life through greater autonomy and convenience in managing their condition.

Kidney Transplantation

Widely regarded as the premier treatment for end-stage kidney disease, kidney transplantation presents the best prospects for enhanced quality of life and prolonged survival when compared to dialysis. During this procedure, a healthy kidney from either a living or deceased donor is surgically implanted into the recipient's body. Subsequently, the transplanted kidney assumes the role of the failed kidneys, effectively restoring kidney function and obviating the necessity for dialysis.

Kidney transplantation boasts several advantages over dialysis:
- **Enhanced quality of life:** Individuals who have undergone kidney transplant procedures frequently express notable enhancements in their overall quality of life. These improvements typically manifest in various aspects, including heightened levels of energy, a revitalized appetite, and an expanded sense of freedom in performing daily activities. Comparatively, when contrasted with individuals undergoing dialysis treatments, transplant recipients often report a significant increase in their physical vitality, a renewed zest for life, and a newfound ability to engage more fully in their daily routines and leisure pursuits. This transformation not only reflects the physiological benefits of transplantation but also underscores the profound impact it can have on one's well-being, providing a testament to the transformative power of medical advancements in

improving the lives of those afflicted with renal conditions.

- **Long-term survival:** Research findings suggest that individuals who have undergone kidney transplantation tend to demonstrate notably higher rates of long-term survival when contrasted with those undergoing regular dialysis treatments. These studies highlight a compelling trend wherein transplant recipients typically experience a prolonged lifespan and enhanced overall health outcomes over extended periods. This advantageous trajectory in survival rates underscores the enduring benefits of kidney transplantation as a preferred treatment modality for individuals with renal disorders. Furthermore, these findings underscore the significance of transplantation not only in extending life expectancy but also in improving the quality of life for patients, offering a promising outlook for those navigating the complexities of renal disease management.

- **Reduced healthcare expenditures:** While kidney transplantation initially involves substantial financial investments, it often emerges as a more economically advantageous option in the long term when compared to the ongoing expenses associated with dialysis, which necessitates continuous treatment and monitoring. Despite the initial financial outlay required for transplantation, the comprehensive analysis of healthcare expenditures reveals a compelling narrative wherein the economic benefits of transplantation become increasingly apparent over time. This shift in cost-effectiveness can be attributed to various factors, including the reduction in recurrent dialysis sessions and related medical interventions, as well as the mitigation of long-term complications associated with renal failure. By minimizing the need for ongoing medical interventions and hospitalizations, kidney transplantation not only presents a more sustainable financial model for healthcare systems but also underscores the significant cost savings and economic efficiencies that can be achieved through prioritizing transplantation as the preferred treatment option for individuals with end-stage renal disease.

Nevertheless, kidney transplantation is not devoid of risks, including the potential for organ rejection and the necessity for lifelong immunosuppressive medications to avert rejection. Furthermore, a scarcity of donor organs results in protracted waiting periods for transplantation.

Palliative Care for End-Stage Kidney Disease

Palliative care is centered on alleviating symptoms and enhancing the quality of life for individuals grappling with severe illnesses such as end-stage kidney disease. The primary objectives of palliative care include addressing physical, emotional, and spiritual needs, thereby assisting patients and their families in navigating the tribulations associated with advanced illness.

Palliative care for end-stage kidney disease encompasses:
- **Symptom management:** The dedicated efforts of palliative care teams are directed towards addressing a spectrum of distressing symptoms frequently encountered by individuals grappling with end-stage kidney disease. These symptoms, encompassing but not limited to pain, nausea, fatigue, and shortness of breath, are central concerns in the holistic management of patients navigating the complexities of advanced renal

illness. By adopting a multidimensional approach, palliative care practitioners prioritize the mitigation of these distressing symptoms, aiming not only to alleviate physical discomfort but also to enhance the overall quality of life for patients and their families. Through personalized interventions tailored to individual needs and preferences, palliative care teams offer a comprehensive continuum of support, encompassing symptom management, psychosocial support, and spiritual care. This integrated approach not only addresses the immediate symptomatic concerns but also fosters a sense of empowerment and well-being among patients, facilitating a more dignified and compassionate journey through the challenges posed by end-stage kidney disease.

- **Emotional support:** Within the realm of palliative care, healthcare providers extend a multifaceted array of services aimed at bolstering emotional well-being and fostering resilience in both patients and their familial support networks as they navigate the complexities inherent in chronic illness. This encompassing approach encompasses not only the provision of counseling and emotional support but also the delivery of tailored guidance and empathetic engagement to assist individuals and their loved ones in confronting and effectively managing the myriad challenges associated with prolonged illness trajectories. Through compassionate and individualized interventions, palliative care practitioners endeavor to create a supportive environment wherein patients and their families feel empowered to navigate the emotional upheavals and uncertainties that often accompany chronic illness with a sense of equanimity and dignity. This collaborative journey towards emotional well-being is characterized by a profound commitment to holistic care, wherein the emotional, psychological, and spiritual dimensions of the human experience are accorded equal importance alongside the management of physical symptoms, ultimately fostering a more comprehensive and compassionate approach to healthcare delivery.

- **Advance care planning:** Palliative care professionals play a pivotal role in facilitating advance care planning, a dynamic process that entails collaboratively assisting patients in articulating their preferences and values regarding various aspects of their healthcare journey, particularly as it pertains to end-of-life care and the formulation of advance directives. This intricate process involves comprehensive discussions that delve into the nuanced intricacies of individual beliefs, desires, and personal priorities, empowering patients to actively engage in decision-making processes that align with their unique needs and aspirations. Through a holistic and person-centered approach, palliative care teams offer a supportive framework wherein patients are encouraged to explore and reflect upon the full spectrum of care options available to them, including potential interventions, treatment modalities, and considerations for end-of-life scenarios. By fostering open and empathetic dialogue, palliative care practitioners facilitate a collaborative journey of self-discovery and empowerment, wherein patients and their loved ones are empowered to make informed decisions that resonate with their values and preferences, ultimately paving the way for a more dignified and personalized healthcare experience.

- **Spiritual care:** Within the holistic framework of palliative care, healthcare providers offer a comprehensive array of services aimed at addressing the spiritual and existential dimensions of patients' experiences, acknowledging and honoring the intricate interplay between belief systems, values, and individual identity. This encompassing approach to spiritual care transcends conventional medical boundaries, embracing a nuanced understanding of human spirituality and existentialism as integral components of the healing process. Through empathetic engagement and culturally sensitive practices, palliative care practitioners create a nurturing environment wherein patients are encouraged to explore and articulate their spiritual beliefs, existential concerns, and profound questions regarding meaning and purpose in the face of illness and mortality. Drawing upon a diverse repertoire of spiritual and religious traditions, as well as non-religious philosophies, these caregivers offer tailored interventions and supportive interventions designed to provide solace, comfort, and meaning in accordance with patients' unique spiritual and existential orientations. By cultivating a space of compassion and understanding, palliative care teams facilitate a transformative journey of self-discovery and spiritual growth, wherein patients and their families find solace, strength, and resilience in the midst of life's most profound challenges.

Palliative care can be delivered alongside curative treatments like dialysis or kidney transplantation or can serve as the principal focus of care for patients either ineligible for or opting against aggressive treatments.

In summary, advanced treatment modalities for Chronic Kidney Disease encompass hemodialysis, peritoneal dialysis, kidney transplantation, and palliative care for individuals with end-stage kidney disease. Each treatment avenue harbors its own advantages and considerations, with the choice of treatment contingent upon individual factors such as disease severity, overall health, and patient preferences. Through a comprehensive understanding of available treatment options and close collaboration with healthcare providers, patients grappling with advanced kidney disease can make informed decisions about their care, thereby optimizing their quality of life.

7: MANAGING COMPLICATIONS OF CHRONIC KIDNEY DISEASE

Delving into the multifaceted realm of managing complications stemming from Chronic Kidney Disease (CKD) is paramount in optimizing patient outcomes and fostering comprehensive well-being. This segment intricately explores a spectrum of strategies aimed at effectively addressing the prevalent complications intertwined with CKD, encompassing a broad range of medical interventions and holistic approaches. Among the pivotal areas of focus are the nuanced management of hypertension and cardiovascular disorders, the intricate navigation of anemia and skeletal abnormalities, and the meticulous balancing act required in addressing electrolyte imbalances and optimizing fluid status. Through a multidisciplinary lens, healthcare professionals delve into the complexities of CKD-related complications, deploying a comprehensive toolkit of therapeutic modalities, lifestyle modifications, and patient-centered interventions tailored to the unique needs and circumstances of each individual. By embracing a holistic approach that extends beyond conventional medical paradigms, practitioners endeavor to empower patients in their journey towards optimal health and well-being, fostering resilience, and promoting a sense of empowerment amidst the challenges posed by CKD and its associated complications.

Hypertension and Cardiovascular Disease

High blood pressure, or hypertension, is both a contributor to and a consequence of CKD, exacerbating kidney damage and elevating the risk of cardiovascular issues. Successfully managing hypertension and cardiovascular disease in CKD patients necessitates a holistic approach involving lifestyle modifications and pharmacotherapy:

1. Blood Pressure Regulation: Regulating blood pressure effectively stands as a cornerstone in the comprehensive management of Chronic Kidney Disease (CKD), with a targeted goal of maintaining levels below 130/80 mmHg deemed pivotal. This intricate facet of CKD care underscores the importance of implementing a multifaceted approach that encompasses not only pharmacological interventions but also lifestyle modifications aimed at optimizing blood pressure control. Encouraging patients to embark on a journey of lifestyle adjustments emerges as a fundamental aspect of this strategy, encompassing a diverse array of tailored recommendations designed to foster blood pressure reduction and overall cardiovascular health. Among these recommendations, advocating for the adoption of a low-sodium diet, the incorporation of regular physical activity into daily routines, and the moderation of alcohol consumption stand out as pivotal pillars in promoting optimal blood pressure regulation. By embracing a holistic paradigm that addresses the interconnectedness of lifestyle factors and cardiovascular health, healthcare providers aim to empower patients in their quest for blood pressure management, fostering a collaborative partnership that underscores the intrinsic link between lifestyle choices and the attainment of therapeutic goals in CKD care.

2. Medication: In conjunction with implementing lifestyle modifications, pharmacological interventions play a crucial role in the holistic management of blood pressure in individuals with Chronic Kidney Disease (CKD), serving as vital tools in safeguarding renal function and promoting overall cardiovascular health. Among the arsenal of medications commonly utilized for blood pressure management, angiotensin-converting enzyme (ACE) inhibitors and angiotensin II receptor blockers (ARBs) stand out as cornerstone agents, revered for their dual benefits in blood pressure control and renal protection. However, the therapeutic armamentarium extends beyond these agents, encompassing a diverse array of antihypertensive drugs tailored to individual patient needs and clinical circumstances. This expansive pharmacological landscape may include the judicious utilization of beta-blockers, calcium channel blockers, and diuretics, each offering unique mechanisms of action and therapeutic profiles aimed at achieving target blood pressure levels while minimizing adverse effects. By harnessing the synergistic potential of pharmacotherapy alongside lifestyle modifications, healthcare providers embark on a collaborative journey with patients, striving to optimize blood pressure management and mitigate the progression of CKD, thereby enhancing both renal and cardiovascular outcomes in this vulnerable population.

3. Cardiovascular Risk Mitigation: In light of the elevated cardiovascular risk inherent in Chronic Kidney Disease (CKD), the strategic mitigation of modifiable risk factors assumes paramount importance in safeguarding against adverse cardiovascular events. This comprehensive approach to cardiovascular risk reduction encompasses a multifaceted array of interventions aimed at addressing an intricate web of interconnected factors, including but not limited to hypertension, dyslipidemia, diabetes, and smoking. By adopting a holistic perspective, healthcare providers delve into the nuanced complexities of each individual risk factor, tailoring interventions to suit the unique needs and circumstances of each patient. Strategies may encompass the meticulous management of blood pressure through pharmacological and lifestyle interventions, the optimization of lipid profiles via targeted therapies and dietary modifications, the vigilant control of blood glucose levels in diabetic individuals, and the implementation of smoking cessation programs to combat the detrimental effects of tobacco use. Through a collaborative partnership between patients and healthcare professionals, this concerted effort towards cardiovascular risk mitigation seeks to not only reduce the incidence of adverse cardiovascular events but also to promote overall health and well-being in individuals navigating the challenges posed by CKD.

Anemia and Bone Disorders:

Anemia and bone disorders frequently manifest in CKD due to impaired kidney function and disruptions in mineral metabolism. Addressing these complications entails a multifaceted approach involving identification of underlying causes and provision of targeted therapies:

1. Anemia Management: Anemia management represents a critical aspect of care in Chronic Kidney Disease (CKD), marked by a decline in red blood cell count or hemoglobin levels, which frequently manifests through debilitating symptoms such as fatigue and shortness of breath. In addressing this multifaceted challenge, healthcare providers deploy a comprehensive armamentarium of therapeutic strategies aimed at alleviating symptoms and optimizing patient well-being. Central to this approach are erythropoiesis-stimulating agents (ESAs), including erythropoietin and darbepoetin, which are routinely prescribed to stimulate the production of red blood cells, thereby ameliorating anemia-related symptoms and improving overall quality of life. However, the management of anemia in CKD extends beyond ESAs alone, with iron supplementation emerging as a crucial adjunctive therapy aimed at rectifying underlying iron deficiency and augmenting the response to ESAs. This integrated approach underscores the importance of addressing the multifactorial nature of anemia in CKD, encompassing a tailored blend of pharmacological interventions, nutritional support, and patient education aimed at optimizing outcomes and enhancing patient-centered care. Through a collaborative partnership between patients and healthcare providers, the management of anemia in CKD unfolds as a dynamic process guided by the principles of individualized care and holistic wellness, with the ultimate goal of alleviating symptoms, restoring vitality, and fostering resilience in the face of chronic illness.

2. Bone Disorder Management: Managing bone disorders in the context of Chronic Kidney Disease (CKD) involves addressing a complex interplay of factors including abnormalities in mineral metabolism, disruptions in vitamin D metabolism, and the development of secondary hyperparathyroidism. These intricacies underscore the multifaceted nature of bone health management in CKD, necessitating a comprehensive approach that spans pharmacological interventions, nutritional supplementation, and vigilant monitoring of disease progression.

One pivotal aspect of bone disorder management revolves around addressing deficiencies in vitamin D, a key player in calcium homeostasis and bone health. Healthcare providers often prescribe vitamin D supplementation to rectify these deficiencies and optimize bone mineralization processes. Additionally, the use of phosphate binders emerges as a cornerstone strategy aimed at lowering serum phosphate levels, thereby mitigating the risk of mineral imbalances and pathological calcification within the skeletal system.

Furthermore, the management of secondary hyperparathyroidism, a common complication in CKD, requires targeted interventions to regulate parathyroid hormone (PTH) levels and prevent skeletal complications. Pharmacological agents, such as calcimimetics and vitamin D analogs, may be employed to modulate PTH secretion and restore hormonal balance within the body.

Integral to the success of bone disorder management is the implementation of regular monitoring protocols aimed at tracking key indicators of bone health and disease progression. Through comprehensive assessment of bone mineral density, serum calcium, phosphate, and PTH levels, healthcare providers are equipped with valuable insights to guide treatment decisions and optimize therapeutic outcomes in individuals with CKD-related bone disorders.

In essence, the management of bone disorders in CKD represents a multifaceted endeavor that necessitates a holistic approach encompassing targeted interventions, proactive monitoring, and patient-centered care. By addressing the underlying pathophysiological mechanisms and optimizing bone health parameters, healthcare providers strive to mitigate the risk of skeletal complications and enhance overall quality of life for individuals navigating the complexities of CKD.

Electrolyte Imbalance and Fluid Management

Electrolyte imbalance and fluid overload are prevalent in CKD and can precipitate serious complications such as arrhythmias and electrolyte disturbances. Addressing these issues involves vigilant monitoring and appropriate interventions:

1. Sodium and Fluid Control: Ensuring optimal sodium and fluid control emerges as a cornerstone in the comprehensive management of Chronic Kidney Disease (CKD), pivotal in mitigating the risks of fluid overload and hypertension while promoting overall cardiovascular health. This multifaceted approach encompasses a spectrum of interventions aimed at empowering patients to navigate dietary and lifestyle modifications tailored to their individual needs and clinical circumstances.

Central to sodium management strategies is the implementation of dietary sodium restriction, wherein healthcare providers advocate for limiting daily sodium intake to less than 2,300 milligrams per day. This targeted approach not only serves to curtail the risk of fluid retention and hypertension but also fosters a cardiovascular-protective milieu conducive to optimal health outcomes.
In tandem with sodium restriction, the judicious management of fluid intake assumes paramount importance in CKD care. By tailoring fluid intake based on individual fluid balance requirements, healthcare providers strive to strike a delicate equilibrium that prevents the onset of fluid overload while ensuring adequate hydration and renal perfusion. This personalized approach acknowledges the nuanced interplay between fluid dynamics, renal function, and cardiovascular health, thereby empowering patients to make

informed decisions regarding their fluid intake habits.

Moreover, healthcare providers engage in collaborative discussions with patients to explore practical strategies for sodium and fluid control, encompassing dietary modifications, fluid monitoring techniques, and lifestyle adjustments tailored to individual preferences and cultural considerations. Through ongoing education, support, and guidance, patients are empowered to take an active role in managing their sodium and fluid intake, thereby fostering a sense of agency and self-efficacy in navigating the complexities of CKD management.

In essence, sodium and fluid control in CKD represent a multifaceted endeavor that transcends mere dietary restrictions, embracing a holistic approach that emphasizes patient education, personalized interventions, and collaborative decision-making. By integrating sodium and fluid management strategies into the broader framework of CKD care, healthcare providers strive to optimize cardiovascular health, mitigate disease progression, and enhance overall quality of life for individuals grappling with the challenges of renal dysfunction.

2. Potassium and Phosphorus Regulation:

Regulating potassium and phosphorus levels represents a critical aspect of managing Chronic Kidney Disease (CKD), given the frequent occurrence of abnormalities in these electrolytes. This multifaceted challenge necessitates a comprehensive approach that encompasses dietary modifications, pharmacological interventions, and close monitoring to achieve optimal electrolyte balance and mitigate associated complications.

Central to potassium and phosphorus regulation strategies is the implementation of targeted dietary modifications aimed at limiting the intake of high-potassium and high-phosphorus foods. Healthcare providers typically advise patients to adopt a balanced diet that prioritizes nutrient-dense, low-potassium, and low-phosphorus options while minimizing the consumption of processed and potassium/phosphorus-rich foods. By empowering patients with practical dietary guidance and meal planning strategies, healthcare providers strive to facilitate adherence to dietary restrictions and promote optimal electrolyte management.

In addition to dietary modifications, pharmacological interventions play a crucial role in addressing electrolyte imbalances in CKD. Healthcare providers may prescribe potassium binders to reduce serum potassium levels and mitigate the risk of hyperkalemia, while phosphate binders serve to lower serum phosphorus levels and minimize the risk of hyperphosphatemia. These pharmacological agents function by binding to excess potassium and phosphorus in the gastrointestinal tract, thereby facilitating their excretion and restoring electrolyte balance.

Furthermore, close monitoring of potassium and phosphorus levels through routine laboratory assessments enables healthcare providers to tailor interventions and adjust treatment regimens based on individual patient needs and disease progression. By leveraging a proactive approach to electrolyte management, healthcare providers strive to optimize clinical outcomes, prevent complications, and enhance overall quality of life for individuals navigating the complexities of CKD.

In essence, potassium and phosphorus regulation in CKD represent multifaceted endeavors that require a collaborative and integrated approach encompassing dietary modifications, pharmacological interventions, and ongoing monitoring. Through comprehensive care coordination and patient education, healthcare providers endeavor to empower individuals with CKD to effectively manage electrolyte imbalances and promote long-term renal health and well-being.

3. Acid-Base Balance: Maintaining proper acid-base balance is crucial in managing the complexities of Chronic Kidney Disease (CKD), as disruptions in this equilibrium can often lead to the development of metabolic acidosis. This intricate interplay of physiological processes underscores the importance of adopting targeted treatment strategies aimed at restoring acid-base homeostasis and optimizing patient outcomes. One common complication encountered in CKD is metabolic acidosis, characterized by a decline in serum bicarbonate levels and an imbalance in acid-base equilibrium. In addressing this challenge, healthcare providers may implement therapeutic interventions centered around bicarbonate supplementation, with the aim of replenishing bicarbonate stores and maintaining serum bicarbonate levels within the physiological range.

Bicarbonate supplementation serves as a cornerstone approach in the management of metabolic acidosis, offering a direct mechanism for neutralizing excess acid and restoring alkaline balance within the body. By administering exogenous bicarbonate, healthcare providers strive to mitigate the deleterious effects of acidosis on various organ systems, including the kidneys, bones, and cardiovascular system, while simultaneously addressing associated symptoms and improving overall patient well-being. Moreover, the management of acid-base balance in CKD extends beyond mere pharmacological interventions, encompassing a holistic approach that considers the underlying pathophysiological mechanisms driving metabolic acidosis. Healthcare providers engage in collaborative discussions with patients to explore potential contributing factors such as dietary habits, medication use, and comorbid conditions, thereby tailoring treatment regimens to address the unique needs and circumstances of each individual. Through comprehensive monitoring and regular assessment of acid-base status, healthcare providers are empowered to make informed decisions regarding treatment adjustments and ongoing management strategies, thereby optimizing clinical outcomes and promoting renal health in individuals with CKD-induced metabolic acidosis.

In essence, the management of acid-base balance in CKD represents a multifaceted endeavor that necessitates a comprehensive understanding of underlying pathophysiology, personalized treatment approaches, and proactive monitoring. By adopting a collaborative and integrative approach to care, healthcare providers strive to restore acid-base homeostasis, alleviate symptoms, and enhance overall quality of life for individuals grappling with the challenges of CKD.

In conclusion, effectively managing complications of Chronic Kidney Disease necessitates a comprehensive approach encompassing hypertension and cardiovascular disease, anemia and bone disorders, and electrolyte imbalance and fluid management. By implementing tailored interventions like lifestyle adjustments, medications, and dietary modifications, healthcare providers can optimize patient outcomes and enhance the quality of life for CKD individuals. Regular monitoring and proactive management of complications are crucial in mitigating disease progression and fostering long-term well-being in CKD patients.

8: LIVING WELL WITH CHRONIC KIDNEY DISEASE

Living with Chronic Kidney Disease (CKD) can be challenging, but with the appropriate strategies and support, individuals can still lead fulfilling lives while managing their condition. This chapter delves into coping mechanisms and emotional assistance, sustaining a high quality of life, and accessing support resources to aid individuals in navigating life with CKD.

Coping Strategies and Emotional Support

1. Education and Knowledge: Encouraging individuals diagnosed with Chronic Kidney Disease (CKD) to actively engage in education and knowledge acquisition is paramount, as access to information serves as a powerful tool for empowerment and self-advocacy. By proactively seeking out resources and information pertaining to their condition, treatment modalities, and lifestyle modifications, individuals with CKD can gain a deeper understanding of their health status and become active participants in their own care journey.

This educational journey extends beyond mere awareness to encompass a comprehensive exploration of CKD and its multifaceted management strategies. Healthcare providers play a pivotal role in facilitating this process by providing accessible and culturally sensitive educational materials, engaging in open and transparent communication, and fostering a collaborative partnership with patients and their families.

By arming themselves with knowledge about CKD, individuals are better equipped to make informed decisions regarding their treatment options, dietary choices, and lifestyle modifications. This proactive approach not only empowers patients to take control of their health but also instills a sense of confidence and self-efficacy in managing the complexities of CKD.

Moreover, understanding CKD and its management can serve as a powerful antidote to anxiety and uncertainty, offering a sense of clarity and direction amidst the challenges posed by chronic illness. By demystifying CKD and providing individuals with the tools and resources they need to navigate their health journey, healthcare providers foster resilience and promote a sense of empowerment in those affected by this condition.

In essence, education and knowledge serve as transformative agents in the realm of CKD management, offering individuals the opportunity to take an active role in their own care, alleviate anxiety, and cultivate a sense of control over their health and well-being. By embracing a collaborative approach that prioritizes education and empowerment, healthcare providers pave the way for enhanced patient outcomes and improved quality of life for individuals living with CKD.

2. Building a Support Network: Building a strong support network is an indispensable aspect of navigating the challenges associated with Chronic Kidney Disease (CKD). Encouraging individuals to cultivate a multifaceted support system can serve as a cornerstone in promoting resilience, fostering emotional well-being, and enhancing overall quality of life amidst the complexities of CKD management.

This endeavor encompasses a comprehensive exploration of various avenues for support, ranging from familial and social networks to formal support groups and online communities. By actively seeking out sources of support, individuals with CKD can access a diverse array of resources and interpersonal connections aimed at providing emotional solace, practical guidance, and encouragement throughout their health journey.

Within the familial and social sphere, individuals are encouraged to lean on loved ones, friends, and caregivers for emotional support, companionship, and assistance with daily tasks. These trusted relationships serve as pillars of strength, offering a safe space for individuals to express their concerns, fears, and triumphs, while also receiving practical assistance and encouragement in navigating the challenges of CKD.

In addition to familial and social networks, formal support groups represent invaluable resources for individuals with CKD seeking solidarity, understanding, and camaraderie from peers facing similar experiences. Participating in support groups facilitates shared experiences, mutual encouragement, and the exchange of practical tips and coping strategies, thereby fostering a sense of community and empowerment among members.

Furthermore, the advent of online communities and virtual support platforms has revolutionized the landscape of CKD support, offering individuals the opportunity to connect with peers, access educational resources, and engage in discussions from the comfort of their own homes. By leveraging the power of technology, individuals can forge meaningful connections, access timely information, and find solace in the shared experiences of others navigating the complexities of CKD.

In essence, building a robust support network is a multifaceted endeavor that requires proactive engagement, openness to vulnerability, and a willingness to seek out and accept support from various sources. By cultivating a diverse support system encompassing familial, social, formal, and virtual networks, individuals with CKD can embark on their health journey with confidence, resilience, and a sense of communal belonging.

3. Effective Communication: Facilitating effective communication between individuals with Chronic Kidney Disease (CKD) and their healthcare providers stands as a fundamental pillar in optimizing patient care and promoting holistic well-being. Encouraging individuals to cultivate an environment of openness and transparency fosters a collaborative partnership wherein concerns can be voiced, questions can be asked, and treatment decisions can be made in a shared decision-making framework.

This multifaceted approach to communication encompasses a spectrum of strategies aimed at empowering individuals to actively engage in their own healthcare journey. By fostering a culture of empowerment and agency, individuals are encouraged to articulate their concerns, express their preferences, and actively participate in treatment discussions, thereby playing an active role in shaping their own care plan.

Furthermore, clear and transparent communication serves as a catalyst for building trust and rapport between individuals and their healthcare providers. By fostering an atmosphere of trust and mutual respect, individuals feel empowered to share their experiences, express their concerns, and collaborate with healthcare providers in devising personalized treatment strategies tailored to their unique needs and circumstances.

In addition to enhancing treatment adherence and promoting positive health outcomes, effective communication serves as a conduit for addressing psychosocial concerns, alleviating anxiety, and fostering a sense of emotional well-being. By providing individuals with the opportunity to voice their fears, uncertainties, and aspirations, healthcare providers can offer reassurance, guidance, and support, thereby promoting resilience and emotional healing amidst the challenges posed by CKD.

In essence, effective communication represents a cornerstone in the holistic management of CKD, offering individuals the opportunity to voice their concerns, engage in shared decision-making, and actively participate in their own care journey. By fostering a culture of openness, transparency, and collaboration, healthcare providers empower individuals to take ownership of their health, promote self-efficacy, and enhance overall well-being in the face of chronic illness.

4. Stress Management Techniques: Coping with the challenges of living with a chronic illness can often entail navigating various stressors that impact overall well-being. In light of this, it is imperative to encourage individuals to proactively incorporate stress management techniques into their daily routines, thereby fostering resilience and promoting a sense of calm amidst the tumultuous landscape of chronic illness.

This multifaceted approach to stress management encompasses a diverse array of techniques and practices aimed at mitigating stressors, alleviating anxiety, and promoting relaxation. By empowering individuals to explore and integrate these techniques into their lifestyle, healthcare providers play a pivotal role in supporting holistic well-being and enhancing coping mechanisms in the face of adversity.

Mindfulness emerges as a central tenet in stress management, encouraging individuals to cultivate present-moment awareness and embrace a non-judgmental attitude towards their thoughts, emotions, and experiences. Through mindfulness practices such as meditation, individuals can develop greater resilience to stress, enhance emotional regulation, and cultivate a deeper sense of inner peace and acceptance.
Additionally, incorporating deep breathing exercises into one's daily routine serves as a powerful tool for reducing stress and promoting relaxation. By engaging in rhythmic breathing patterns and focusing on the breath, individuals can activate the body's natural relaxation response, thereby reducing tension, calming the mind, and restoring equilibrium amidst the challenges of chronic illness.

Moreover, the practice of yoga represents a holistic approach to stress management that integrates physical postures, breathwork, and mindfulness techniques to promote overall well-being. Through regular practice, individuals can experience enhanced flexibility, strength, and balance, while also cultivating a sense of inner calm, resilience, and self-awareness.

In essence, embracing stress management techniques represents a proactive and empowering approach to coping with the challenges of living with a chronic illness. By encouraging individuals to explore and integrate mindfulness, meditation, deep breathing exercises, and yoga into their daily routines, healthcare providers empower individuals to cultivate resilience, promote relaxation, and enhance overall quality of life amidst the complexities of chronic illness.

Maintaining Quality of Life

1. Nutrition Focus: Fostering a nutritionally sound diet serves as a cornerstone in the comprehensive management of Chronic Kidney Disease (CKD), facilitating the maintenance of overall health and well-being. Encouraging individuals to adhere to personalized dietary recommendations provided by healthcare providers forms an integral aspect of this endeavor, as it empowers individuals to make informed choices that support renal health and optimize nutritional status.

Central to this approach is the emphasis on dietary modifications aimed at addressing specific nutrient considerations commonly encountered in CKD, including restrictions on sodium, potassium, phosphorus, and protein intake. By advocating for adherence to these dietary guidelines, healthcare providers equip individuals with the knowledge and tools necessary to mitigate the risk of electrolyte imbalances, minimize renal workload, and prevent the progression of kidney disease.

Furthermore, promoting portion control and meal planning emerges as pivotal strategies in fostering adherence to dietary recommendations and achieving nutritional goals. By encouraging individuals to adopt mindful eating practices, healthcare providers facilitate greater awareness of portion sizes, food choices, and meal composition, thereby empowering individuals to make conscious decisions that align with their nutritional needs and health objectives.

Moreover, regular monitoring of nutritional status serves as a proactive approach to assessing dietary adequacy, identifying potential deficiencies or imbalances, and guiding adjustments to dietary interventions as needed. Through comprehensive nutritional assessment and ongoing monitoring, healthcare providers can tailor dietary recommendations to address evolving nutritional needs and optimize health outcomes in individuals with CKD.

In essence, focusing on nutrition represents a holistic approach to CKD management that encompasses dietary modifications, portion control, meal planning, and regular nutritional status monitoring. By fostering a collaborative partnership between individuals and healthcare providers, this approach empowers individuals to take an active role in their own nutritional health, promote renal function, and enhance overall well-being amidst the challenges of chronic kidney disease.

2. Staying Active: Promoting a lifestyle of regular physical activity holds significant merit for individuals grappling with Chronic Kidney Disease (CKD), as it encompasses a myriad of benefits spanning cardiovascular health enhancement, maintenance of muscle strength, and overall enhancement of quality of life. Encouraging individuals to integrate physical activity into their daily routine emerges as a pivotal strategy in fostering resilience, promoting well-being, and mitigating the impact of CKD on physical function and vitality.

Embracing a holistic approach to physical activity entails advocating for participation in a diverse array of enjoyable and accessible activities tailored to individual preferences and capabilities. Whether it be leisurely walks in the park, invigorating swims in the pool, leisurely cycling outings, or engaging in low-impact exercises, the emphasis lies on finding activities that resonate with personal interests while considering any physical limitations or restrictions.

Furthermore, highlighting the multifaceted benefits of physical activity serves to underscore its intrinsic value in CKD management. Beyond the tangible improvements in cardiovascular health and muscle strength, regular physical activity fosters a sense of empowerment, resilience, and emotional well-being, thereby enhancing overall quality of life for individuals navigating the complexities of chronic illness.

Moreover, acknowledging and addressing potential barriers to physical activity, such as physical limitations, comorbidities, or logistical challenges, is paramount in facilitating successful adherence to an active lifestyle. By collaborating with healthcare providers to develop personalized exercise plans and implementing strategies to overcome obstacles, individuals can cultivate sustainable habits that promote long-term health and vitality.

In essence, staying active represents a proactive and empowering approach to CKD management, offering individuals the opportunity to reclaim agency over their health, promote physical function, and enhance overall well-being. By advocating for regular physical activity participation, healthcare providers empower individuals to embrace a lifestyle of vitality, resilience, and holistic wellness amidst the challenges posed by chronic kidney disease.

3. Medication Management: Effectively managing medications plays a pivotal role in navigating the complexities of Chronic Kidney Disease (CKD) and mitigating the risk of associated complications. Encouraging individuals to prioritize consistency and adherence in their medication routines emerges as a cornerstone in promoting optimal health outcomes and enhancing overall well-being amidst the challenges posed by CKD.

Central to medication management is the cultivation of a proactive and vigilant approach towards adherence, wherein individuals are empowered to take ownership of their medication regimens and prioritize adherence to prescribed treatment protocols. This entails fostering a mindset of accountability and responsibility, wherein individuals are encouraged to take medications as directed, adhere to prescribed dosages, and adhere to prescribed schedules with unwavering consistency.

Furthermore, fostering open lines of communication between individuals and their healthcare team serves as a vital component in medication management, facilitating the exchange of information, addressing concerns, and monitoring for potential side effects or adverse reactions. By encouraging individuals to communicate openly and transparently with their healthcare providers, barriers to adherence can be identified and addressed proactively, thereby enhancing treatment efficacy and optimizing therapeutic outcomes.

Moreover, fostering a collaborative partnership between individuals and their healthcare providers is essential in navigating the complexities of medication management in CKD. By engaging in shared decision-making processes, individuals are empowered to actively participate in treatment decisions, voice concerns, and collaborate with their healthcare team to tailor medication regimens to their unique needs and circumstances.

In essence, medication management represents a multifaceted endeavor that requires a holistic approach encompassing adherence, communication, and collaboration. By empowering individuals to prioritize consistency in medication adherence, communicate openly with their healthcare providers, and actively engage in shared decision-making processes, healthcare providers foster a culture of empowerment, accountability, and proactive health management in individuals grappling with the challenges of CKD.

4. Addressing Mental Health: Navigating the journey of Chronic Kidney Disease (CKD) can exert significant strain on mental health, underscoring the importance of prioritizing emotional well-being and fostering resilience amidst the challenges posed by chronic illness. Encouraging individuals to proactively address their mental health needs serves as a cornerstone in promoting holistic wellness and enhancing overall quality of life.

Central to this approach is the recognition of mental health as a vital component of comprehensive CKD management, warranting attention, and prioritization alongside physical health concerns. By fostering a culture of openness and stigmatization surrounding mental health, individuals are empowered to recognize and address their emotional needs in a proactive and supportive environment.

One avenue for addressing mental health concerns is through seeking support from mental health professionals, such as therapists or counselors, who possess the expertise and resources to provide tailored interventions and support strategies. By engaging in therapy or counseling, individuals can explore coping mechanisms, develop resilience, and cultivate adaptive strategies for managing stress, anxiety, and depression associated with CKD.

Moreover, promoting self-care routines that prioritize relaxation and emotional well-being serves as a proactive approach to enhancing mental health outcomes in individuals with CKD. Encouraging individuals to integrate self-care practices such as mindfulness, meditation, journaling, or engaging in hobbies and leisure activities that bring joy and fulfillment can foster a sense of balance, resilience, and emotional equilibrium amidst the challenges of chronic illness.

Furthermore, fostering a supportive environment that encourages open communication and validation of emotional experiences is essential in promoting mental well-being in individuals with

CKD. By creating spaces for individuals to express their concerns, fears, and uncertainties without judgment, healthcare providers foster a sense of belonging, understanding, and validation, thereby promoting emotional healing and resilience in the face of adversity.

In essence, addressing mental health concerns in individuals with CKD represents a multifaceted endeavor that requires a comprehensive and holistic approach encompassing support from mental health professionals, engagement in therapy or counseling, adoption of self-care practices, and fostering a supportive environment that validates emotional experiences. By prioritizing mental well-being alongside physical health concerns, individuals can cultivate resilience, promote emotional well-being, and enhance overall quality of life amidst the challenges of living with CKD.

Accessing Support Resources

1. Patient Education Programs: Patient education programs tailored for individuals with Chronic Kidney Disease (CKD) are widely available across various healthcare institutions and organizations. These programs serve as invaluable resources, offering a wealth of information, support, and practical guidance to empower individuals in navigating the complexities of their condition and enhancing their ability to manage it effectively.

Central to the ethos of these patient education programs is the recognition of the unique challenges and needs faced by individuals with CKD. By tailoring educational content and resources to address the specific concerns and circumstances of this population, healthcare providers strive to equip individuals with the knowledge, skills, and confidence necessary to make informed decisions about their health and well-being.

These programs encompass a diverse array of educational modalities, ranging from structured classes and workshops to individualized counseling sessions and online resources. By offering flexibility in delivery formats, patient education programs cater to the diverse learning preferences and accessibility needs of individuals with CKD, ensuring that information and support are accessible to all.

Moreover, patient education programs serve as a hub for fostering peer support and community engagement, providing individuals with opportunities to connect with others facing similar challenges, share experiences, and exchange insights and coping strategies. Through these collaborative interactions, individuals with CKD can draw strength, validation, and encouragement from their peers, fostering a sense of camaraderie and belonging amidst the journey of chronic illness.

Furthermore, the ongoing evolution of patient education programs reflects a commitment to continuous improvement and responsiveness to the evolving needs of individuals with CKD. By soliciting feedback, incorporating evidence-based practices, and adapting content to reflect emerging research and clinical guidelines, healthcare providers ensure that patient education programs remain relevant, impactful, and responsive to the ever-changing landscape of CKD management.

In essence, patient education programs represent a cornerstone in the comprehensive care of individuals with CKD, offering a multifaceted approach to empowerment, support, and education.

By leveraging these resources, individuals can enhance their knowledge, cultivate self-efficacy, and optimize their ability to manage their condition effectively, thereby promoting better health outcomes and enhancing overall quality of life amidst the challenges of living with CKD.

2. Support Groups: Engaging in support groups tailored for individuals grappling with Chronic Kidney Disease (CKD) provides a vital avenue for fostering a supportive community, cultivating empathy, and offering mutual encouragement. These support networks serve as invaluable platforms, offering a multitude of opportunities for individuals to connect, share their journeys, and draw strength from the collective wisdom and experiences of their peers navigating similar challenges associated with CKD.

Central to the ethos of support groups is the recognition of the unique emotional and practical needs of individuals living with CKD. By providing a safe and empathetic space for individuals to express their concerns, fears, and triumphs, support groups foster a sense of camaraderie and solidarity, offering validation, understanding, and encouragement to those grappling with the complexities of chronic illness.

Participation in support groups offers individuals the opportunity to gain insights, perspectives, and coping strategies from others who intimately understand the intricacies of living with CKD. Through shared experiences, individuals can glean valuable wisdom, practical tips, and emotional support, thereby enhancing their ability to navigate the challenges of CKD with resilience and fortitude.

Moreover, support groups serve as hubs for information exchange and resource sharing, offering individuals access to a wealth of educational materials, expert insights, and community-driven initiatives aimed at empowering individuals to make informed decisions about their health and well-being.

Furthermore, support groups foster a culture of empathy and compassion, wherein individuals feel seen, heard, and valued for their unique experiences and perspectives. By fostering a sense of belonging and validation, support groups promote emotional healing, resilience, and empowerment in individuals grappling with the psychosocial impacts of CKD.

In essence, participation in support groups represents a transformative journey of connection, growth, and healing for individuals living with CKD. By embracing the support and camaraderie of peers, individuals can find solace, strength, and hope amidst the challenges of chronic illness, ultimately fostering a sense of community, understanding, and encouragement that transcends the boundaries of disease.

3. Online Resources: The vast expanse of the internet offers a treasure trove of invaluable resources and information tailored specifically for individuals grappling with Chronic Kidney Disease (CKD) and their caregivers. Encouraging individuals to embark on a journey of exploration through reputable online platforms, including dedicated websites, forums, and social media groups focused on CKD, presents an opportunity for knowledge acquisition, connection-building, and accessing much-needed support in navigating the complexities of the condition.

Central to this endeavor is the recognition of the internet as a dynamic and ever-expanding repository of knowledge, where individuals can embark on a quest for information, insights, and resources that cater to their unique needs and circumstances. By encouraging individuals to explore reputable websites curated by trusted healthcare organizations, advocacy groups, and reputable medical institutions, healthcare providers empower individuals to access accurate, up-to-date information on CKD management, treatment options, and lifestyle recommendations. Moreover, online forums and social media groups dedicated to CKD offer a virtual space for individuals to connect, share experiences, and exchange insights with others who are facing similar challenges. By fostering a sense of community, camaraderie, and understanding, these online platforms provide a lifeline of support and encouragement to individuals navigating the ups and downs of life with CKD, fostering a sense of belonging and validation amidst the journey of chronic illness.

Furthermore, online resources serve as a gateway to empowerment and self-advocacy, enabling individuals to become informed advocates for their own health and well-being. By providing access to a wealth of educational materials, peer-reviewed articles, and expert insights, online platforms empower individuals to make informed decisions about their care, engage in meaningful discussions with healthcare providers, and advocate for their needs within the healthcare system.

In essence, embracing online resources represents a transformative journey of empowerment, connection, and self-discovery for individuals living with CKD and their caregivers. By encouraging exploration of reputable online platforms, healthcare providers facilitate access to a wealth of information, support, and community that can enrich the lives of individuals affected by CKD, ultimately fostering resilience, empowerment, and a renewed sense of hope amidst the challenges of chronic illness.

4. Healthcare Navigation Services: Traversing the intricate labyrinth of the healthcare system, particularly for individuals grappling with multifaceted medical conditions such as Chronic Kidney Disease (CKD), can often feel like embarking on a daunting journey fraught with challenges and uncertainties. In recognition of this reality, healthcare navigation services emerge as invaluable allies, offering a guiding hand and a beacon of support to individuals and their caregivers as they navigate the complexities of the healthcare landscape.

At the heart of healthcare navigation services lies a commitment to empowering individuals and caregivers with the knowledge, resources, and support necessary to navigate the intricacies of the healthcare system with confidence and ease. By serving as knowledgeable guides and advocates, healthcare navigators offer personalized assistance tailored to the unique needs and circumstances of each individual, ensuring that no stone is left unturned in the quest for optimal care and support.

One of the primary roles of healthcare navigation services is to assist individuals and caregivers in accessing and understanding the myriad resources available within the healthcare system. From identifying appropriate healthcare providers and specialists to facilitating access to diagnostic tests, treatments, and support services, healthcare navigators serve as invaluable conduits, streamlining the process of accessing care and ensuring that individuals receive the comprehensive support they need to manage their condition effectively.

Moreover, healthcare navigation services play a vital role in facilitating effective communication and coordination among various healthcare providers involved in the care of individuals with CKD. By serving as liaisons between patients, caregivers, and healthcare teams, navigators help bridge gaps in communication, facilitate information sharing, and ensure that everyone involved in the care continuum is aligned and working collaboratively towards shared goals of health and well-being.

Additionally, healthcare navigation services extend beyond the confines of the healthcare system to encompass advocacy, education, and empowerment. By providing individuals and caregivers with the tools, knowledge, and resources to advocate for their own needs within the healthcare system, navigators empower them to become active participants in their care journey, fostering a sense of agency, resilience, and self-advocacy amidst the complexities of managing CKD.

In essence, healthcare navigation services represent a lifeline of support and guidance for individuals and caregivers navigating the intricate terrain of the healthcare system. By offering personalized assistance, advocacy, and empowerment, healthcare navigators empower individuals to navigate the complexities of CKD with confidence, resilience, and a renewed sense of hope for the future.

In summary, living well with Chronic Kidney Disease is attainable with suitable coping strategies, support, and resources. By focusing on emotional well-being, maintaining quality of life, and utilizing support resources, individuals with CKD can effectively manage their condition, enhance their overall well-being, and lead fulfilling lives despite the challenges they may encounter. Encourage individuals to actively engage in their care, seek support when needed, and prioritize self-care to optimize their quality of life with CKD.

9: SPECIAL CONSIDERATIONS IN CHRONIC KIDNEY DISEASE

Chronic Kidney Disease (CKD) poses multifaceted challenges that vary across different age groups and life stages, necessitating tailored approaches for diagnosis, treatment, and management. This segment explores the nuanced considerations inherent in CKD management for individuals at different developmental stages, including children and adolescents, older adults, and pregnant individuals.

CKD manifests uniquely in each age demographic, with distinct clinical presentations, treatment considerations, and prognostic implications. Understanding these nuances is essential for healthcare providers to deliver optimal care that addresses the specific needs and challenges faced by individuals at different stages of life.

In pediatric CKD, early detection and intervention are paramount to mitigate disease progression and optimize long-term outcomes. Children with CKD often present with unique clinical manifestations and developmental considerations, requiring specialized diagnostic approaches, tailored treatment modalities, and comprehensive multidisciplinary care teams to address their complex needs effectively.

Similarly, CKD in older adults presents its own set of challenges, including comorbidities, polypharmacy, and age-related physiological changes that may influence disease progression and treatment outcomes. Healthcare providers must adopt a holistic approach that accounts for the unique health needs and preferences of older adults, while also addressing age-related considerations such as frailty, cognitive impairment, and end-of-life planning.

Pregnant individuals with CKD face additional complexities, as the physiological changes of pregnancy can exacerbate renal dysfunction and increase the risk of complications for both the mother and fetus. Management strategies must balance the need to preserve renal function with the safety of the developing fetus, necessitating close monitoring, collaborative care between nephrologists and obstetricians, and individualized treatment plans tailored to the specific needs of each patient.

In essence, CKD management requires a nuanced understanding of the distinct challenges and considerations present at different stages of life.

By recognizing and addressing these unique factors, healthcare providers can deliver personalized care that optimizes outcomes and enhances quality of life for individuals living with CKD across the lifespan.

CKD in Children and Adolescents

1. Diagnosis Challenges: Diagnosing Chronic Kidney Disease (CKD) in children and adolescents presents a unique set of challenges characterized by diverse symptomatology, variable disease progression, and the dynamic nature of developmental stages. Detecting CKD at an early stage is imperative to preempt potential complications and maximize treatment effectiveness. Within this demographic, pediatricians and pediatric nephrologists assume pivotal roles in recognizing and addressing CKD, underscoring the importance of collaboration and expertise in providing comprehensive care.

The process of identifying CKD in pediatric populations entails navigating a complex landscape shaped by a multitude of factors, including age-specific variations in symptom presentation, physiological maturation, and disease trajectory. Unlike adults, children and adolescents may exhibit atypical or subtle symptoms of CKD, necessitating a high index of suspicion and thorough evaluation by healthcare providers. Moreover, the evolving nature of developmental stages adds another layer of complexity to the diagnostic process, as manifestations of CKD may manifest differently across various age groups and growth phases. Pediatricians and pediatric nephrologists must therefore remain vigilant in recognizing potential signs of CKD, adapting diagnostic approaches to accommodate the unique needs and characteristics of each patient.

Timely detection of CKD is paramount to initiating appropriate interventions and preventing the progression of kidney dysfunction. Pediatricians and pediatric nephrologists collaborate closely to implement screening protocols, interpret diagnostic tests, and monitor renal function over time, thereby facilitating early intervention and optimization of treatment outcomes.

Furthermore, the interdisciplinary nature of pediatric CKD care underscores the importance of a coordinated approach involving various healthcare professionals, including nurses, dietitians, and social workers, to address the multifaceted needs of patients and families. By fostering collaboration and communication among team members, healthcare providers can optimize care delivery and enhance the overall well-being of children and adolescents living with CKD.

In essence, diagnosing CKD in children and adolescents necessitates a comprehensive and multidisciplinary approach that recognizes the unique challenges and complexities inherent in this demographic. By leveraging expertise, collaboration, and a patient-centered mindset, healthcare providers can enhance diagnostic accuracy, promote timely intervention, and improve outcomes for pediatric patients with CKD.

2. Growth and Development: Chronic Kidney Disease (CKD) has the potential to hamper the growth and developmental trajectories of children and adolescents, potentially resulting in delays in physical growth, onset of puberty, and overall developmental milestones. Close monitoring of growth parameters, implementation of tailored nutritional interventions, and consideration of growth hormone therapy represent essential pillars of CKD management in pediatric populations, underscoring the multifaceted approach required to address the complex interplay between renal health and growth dynamics during critical developmental stages.

The impact of CKD on growth and development in pediatric patients underscores the intricate relationship between renal function and physiological maturation. Children and adolescents with CKD may experience disruptions in linear growth, characterized by slower growth rates and diminished stature compared to their peers. Furthermore, impaired kidney function can influence the timing and progression of pubertal development, potentially leading to delayed onset of secondary sexual characteristics and reproductive maturation.

In light of these challenges, vigilant monitoring of growth parameters emerges as a cornerstone in pediatric CKD management, facilitating early detection of growth disturbances and timely intervention to mitigate their impact. Healthcare providers employ a range of anthropometric measurements, including height, weight, and body mass index, to track growth trajectories and identify deviations from expected norms, thereby informing personalized treatment strategies tailored to the unique needs of each patient.

Nutritional support plays a pivotal role in optimizing growth and development in children and adolescents with CKD, addressing both macro- and micronutrient requirements essential for healthy growth. Dietitians collaborate closely with healthcare teams to formulate individualized dietary plans that promote optimal growth while addressing specific dietary restrictions and renal health considerations. Emphasis is placed on adequate protein intake, micronutrient supplementation, and calorie optimization to support energy needs and facilitate growth in pediatric CKD patients.

In cases where growth disturbances persist despite nutritional interventions, consideration may be given to growth hormone therapy as a supplementary treatment modality. Growth hormone supplementation can stimulate linear growth and promote catch-up growth in pediatric patients with CKD, offering a targeted approach to addressing growth deficits and optimizing final adult height.

In essence, addressing growth and developmental challenges in children and adolescents with CKD requires a multifaceted and holistic approach that encompasses close monitoring, nutritional optimization, and consideration of adjunctive therapies. By addressing the unique needs of pediatric patients with CKD, healthcare providers can mitigate the impact of renal dysfunction on growth trajectories, foster optimal development, and improve long-term outcomes for this vulnerable population.

3. Psychosocial Support: Navigating the complexities of Chronic Kidney Disease (CKD) poses significant emotional and social challenges for young individuals, impacting various facets of their lives including emotional well-being, social interactions, and academic pursuits. Recognizing the profound psychosocial implications of CKD on pediatric patients and their families, access to comprehensive psychosocial support services emerges as a critical component in addressing the multifaceted needs of this vulnerable population.

The psychosocial impact of CKD on young individuals extends beyond the physical manifestations of the disease, encompassing a spectrum of emotional, social, and academic concerns that can significantly impact their quality of life and overall well-being. From coping with the emotional turmoil of chronic illness to navigating social dynamics and academic pressures, pediatric patients with CKD face a myriad of challenges that warrant sensitive and comprehensive support interventions.

In response to these challenges, the provision of psychosocial support services tailored to the unique needs of young CKD patients and their families assumes paramount importance. These services encompass a range of interventions aimed at addressing emotional distress, fostering social connectedness, and promoting academic success in the face of adversity.

Counseling services play a central role in providing emotional support and guidance to young CKD patients and their families, offering a safe and confidential space to explore feelings, cope with stressors, and develop adaptive coping strategies. Through individual or family counseling sessions, patients and caregivers can gain valuable insights, enhance communication skills, and strengthen resilience in the face of chronic illness.

In addition to counseling, peer support groups offer a valuable avenue for young CKD patients to connect with peers facing similar challenges, share experiences, and draw strength from collective solidarity. These peer-driven forums provide a sense of belonging, validation, and understanding, fostering a supportive community where individuals can find solace, empathy, and encouragement amidst the complexities of living with CKD.

Furthermore, access to educational resources tailored to the unique needs of young CKD patients and their families serves as a vital tool in promoting understanding, empowerment, and self-management skills. By providing accurate information about CKD, treatment options, and lifestyle management strategies, these resources empower patients and caregivers to make informed decisions, advocate for their needs, and navigate the healthcare system with confidence.

In essence, psychosocial support services represent a cornerstone in pediatric CKD care, offering a holistic approach to addressing the emotional, social, and academic needs of young patients and their families. By providing a comprehensive array of support interventions, healthcare providers can mitigate the psychosocial impact of CKD, enhance resilience, and improve overall quality of life for this vulnerable population.

CKD in Older Adults

1. Aging and Kidney Function: The process of aging entails a multitude of structural and functional alterations in the kidneys, rendering older adults more susceptible to the development of Chronic Kidney Disease (CKD) and its attendant complications. As individuals age, their kidneys undergo gradual changes in size, composition, and function, predisposing them to an elevated risk of CKD and associated comorbidities.

The prevalence of CKD escalates significantly with advancing age, reflecting the cumulative impact of age-related alterations in renal physiology and the increased prevalence of predisposing factors such as hypertension, diabetes, and cardiovascular disease. These concurrent conditions commonly coexist with CKD in older adults, creating a complex interplay of risk factors and comorbidities that can pose formidable challenges for management and treatment.

In addition to age-related changes in kidney structure and function, older adults often present with a constellation of comorbidities and risk factors that further exacerbate the complexity of CKD management. Hypertension, diabetes, and cardiovascular disease are prevalent among older adults and are closely intertwined with CKD pathogenesis, exacerbating renal dysfunction and increasing the risk of adverse outcomes.

Furthermore, the presence of multiple comorbidities in older adults necessitates a comprehensive and multidisciplinary approach to CKD management, wherein healthcare providers must navigate the intricate interplay between various disease processes and treatment modalities. Collaborative efforts between nephrologists, primary care physicians, cardiologists, and other specialists are essential to address the diverse needs of older adults with CKD and mitigate the risk of complications.

Moreover, the management of CKD in older adults must take into account age-related physiological changes, medication-related concerns, and considerations related to functional status and quality of life. Tailoring treatment strategies to align with the individual needs and preferences of older adults, while balancing the risks and benefits of interventions, is paramount to optimizing outcomes and enhancing overall well-being in this demographic.

In essence, aging is intricately linked with alterations in kidney function and structure, predisposing older adults to an increased risk of CKD and its associated complications. Recognizing the unique challenges posed by CKD in older adults, healthcare providers must adopt a holistic and individualized approach to management that addresses the complex interplay of age-related changes, comorbidities, and treatment considerations, thereby promoting optimal outcomes and quality of life in this vulnerable population.

2. Diagnosis and Assessment: The process of diagnosing and evaluating Chronic Kidney Disease (CKD) in older adults requires a meticulous approach that takes into account the unique challenges posed by age-related changes, the presence of comorbidities, and variations in functional status. Given the complexity of CKD presentation in this demographic, it is essential to employ validated assessment tools and guidelines, such as those provided by the Kidney Disease: Improving Global Outcomes (KDIGO), to ensure accurate staging of CKD and inform tailored treatment strategies.

As individuals age, there is a natural progression of physiological changes in kidney function, including alterations in glomerular filtration rate (GFR), renal blood flow, and tubular function. These age-related changes can complicate the diagnosis and assessment of CKD in older adults, necessitating a nuanced understanding of normal aging processes versus pathological changes indicative of CKD.
Furthermore, older adults commonly present with a myriad of comorbidities, such as hypertension, diabetes, and cardiovascular disease, which can influence the clinical presentation and progression

of CKD. The presence of these concurrent conditions adds complexity to the diagnostic process, requiring healthcare providers to carefully consider the interplay between CKD and comorbidities when evaluating older adults with renal impairment.

In addition to age-related alterations and comorbidities, functional status plays a crucial role in the diagnosis and assessment of CKD in older adults. Impairments in functional status, such as reduced mobility, cognitive decline, and frailty, can impact the interpretation of laboratory tests and imaging studies, as well as the feasibility and tolerability of treatment interventions.

To navigate these complexities, healthcare providers rely on validated assessment tools and guidelines, such as the KDIGO guidelines, to standardize the diagnostic process and ensure consistency in CKD staging and management. These guidelines offer evidence-based recommendations for the evaluation of kidney function, assessment of albuminuria, and determination of CKD severity, facilitating a systematic approach to diagnosis and treatment decision-making in older adults.

In summary, diagnosing and assessing CKD in older adults requires a comprehensive understanding of age-related changes, comorbidities, and functional status. By utilizing validated assessment tools and guidelines, healthcare providers can accurately stage CKD, identify appropriate treatment interventions, and optimize outcomes in this vulnerable population.

3. Treatment Challenges: The management of Chronic Kidney Disease (CKD) in older adults presents a multitude of challenges, stemming from various factors including polypharmacy, drug interactions, and age-related alterations in drug metabolism and elimination. Addressing these treatment complexities requires a tailored approach that considers individual patient characteristics, comorbidities, and preferences, with the ultimate goal of optimizing therapeutic outcomes and preserving quality of life in this demographic.

One of the primary challenges encountered in treating CKD in older adults is the prevalence of polypharmacy, wherein patients are prescribed multiple medications to manage various comorbidities and health conditions. This polypharmacy phenomenon increases the risk of adverse drug reactions, drug interactions, and medication non-adherence, thereby complicating the overall management of CKD and contributing to treatment-related challenges.

Moreover, older adults often experience age-related changes in drug metabolism and elimination, resulting in altered pharmacokinetics and increased susceptibility to drug toxicity. Reduced renal function, impaired hepatic metabolism, and alterations in drug distribution and clearance can affect the pharmacological response to medications, necessitating careful dose adjustments and monitoring to ensure safety and efficacy.

Additionally, the presence of multiple comorbidities in older adults further complicates CKD management, as treatment decisions must account for the potential impact of concurrent health conditions on renal function and treatment outcomes. Healthcare providers must strike a delicate balance between managing CKD and addressing other health concerns, prioritizing interventions that optimize overall health and well-being while minimizing the risk of treatment-related complications.

Customizing treatment plans to accommodate medication adjustments, comorbidity management, and individual patient preferences is paramount in optimizing outcomes for older adults with CKD. This may involve simplifying medication regimens, prioritizing medications with proven efficacy and safety profiles, and actively involving patients in shared decision-making processes to ensure alignment with their treatment goals and preferences.

Furthermore, close collaboration between healthcare providers, including nephrologists, primary care physicians, pharmacists, and other specialists, is essential in navigating treatment complexities and coordinating care for older adults with CKD. Multidisciplinary care teams can leverage their collective expertise to address the diverse needs of older adults, optimize medication management, and promote holistic approaches to CKD management that prioritize patient-centered care and quality of life.

In summary, managing CKD in older adults requires a comprehensive and individualized approach that takes into account the unique treatment challenges associated with aging, polypharmacy, and comorbidity burden. By tailoring treatment plans to accommodate these complexities and engaging in collaborative decision-making, healthcare providers can optimize therapeutic outcomes and enhance the overall well-being of older adults with CKD.

CKD and Pregnancy

1. Maternal and Fetal Risks: The presence of Chronic Kidney Disease (CKD) during pregnancy introduces significant complexities and risks, affecting the well-being of both the mother and the developing fetus. Pregnant individuals with CKD are confronted with elevated risks of experiencing a range of complications, including but not limited to preeclampsia, gestational hypertension, preterm birth, fetal growth restriction, and adverse outcomes for both maternal and fetal health. The management of CKD during pregnancy requires diligent oversight and collaboration among a multidisciplinary team consisting of obstetricians, nephrologists, and maternal-fetal medicine specialists, with the primary objective of minimizing risks and optimizing outcomes for both mother and baby.

The interplay between CKD and pregnancy introduces a complex array of challenges and considerations that necessitate comprehensive monitoring and management strategies to mitigate potential risks and ensure the best possible outcomes for all parties involved. Pregnant individuals with CKD are at increased risk of developing hypertensive disorders such as preeclampsia and gestational hypertension, which can have profound implications for maternal health and fetal development. These conditions require vigilant monitoring and early intervention to prevent complications and minimize adverse outcomes.

In addition to hypertensive disorders, CKD during pregnancy is associated with an elevated risk of preterm birth, characterized by the delivery of the baby before 37 weeks of gestation. Preterm birth can lead to a range of health complications for the newborn, including respiratory distress syndrome, feeding difficulties, and long-term developmental challenges. Therefore, careful monitoring and management of CKD-related factors are essential to reduce the risk of preterm birth and optimize neonatal outcomes.

Furthermore, fetal growth restriction, characterized by below-average growth of the fetus, is another potential complication of CKD during pregnancy. Fetal growth restriction can result in low birth weight, increased risk of perinatal complications, and long-term health implications for the baby. Close monitoring of fetal growth and development, along with appropriate interventions to optimize maternal health and fetal nutrition, are crucial to minimizing the risk of fetal growth restriction and promoting healthy outcomes for both mother and baby.

Given the complex nature of CKD during pregnancy and the potential for adverse outcomes, close collaboration among a multidisciplinary team of healthcare providers is indispensable. Obstetricians, nephrologists, and maternal-fetal medicine specialists must work together to develop individualized care plans that address the unique needs and challenges of pregnant individuals with CKD. This collaborative approach allows for comprehensive monitoring, timely interventions, and proactive management of complications, ultimately leading to improved outcomes for both maternal and fetal health.

In summary, CKD complicates pregnancy and poses risks to both maternal and fetal well-being. Close monitoring and collaboration among a multidisciplinary team of healthcare providers are essential to mitigate risks, optimize outcomes, and ensure the best possible care for pregnant individuals with CKD and their babies.

2. Preconception Counseling: Preconception counseling serves as a critical component of care for women of childbearing age who have Chronic Kidney Disease (CKD). It provides an invaluable opportunity to engage in comprehensive discussions about the potential risks and challenges associated with pregnancy, explore available contraceptive options, and address concerns related to fertility preservation for those desiring future pregnancies. By optimizing maternal health, managing underlying comorbidities, and making necessary adjustments to medications prior to conception, healthcare providers can significantly enhance the likelihood of positive pregnancy outcomes while reducing the incidence of maternal and fetal complications.

The process of preconception counseling involves a thorough evaluation of the woman's overall health status, including her kidney function, cardiovascular health, and presence of any other medical conditions or risk factors that may impact pregnancy. This comprehensive assessment allows healthcare providers to identify and address potential barriers to a successful pregnancy, such as uncontrolled hypertension, poorly managed diabetes, or medication regimens that may pose risks to fetal development.

In addition to assessing medical factors, preconception counseling provides an opportunity to discuss lifestyle modifications and behaviors that can optimize maternal health and promote successful pregnancy outcomes. This may include recommendations for maintaining a healthy weight, adopting a balanced diet rich in essential nutrients, engaging in regular physical activity, and avoiding harmful substances such as tobacco, alcohol, and illicit drugs.

Contraceptive counseling is also an integral component of preconception care for women with CKD who are not currently seeking pregnancy. By exploring available contraceptive options and discussing their respective benefits, risks, and effectiveness, healthcare providers can help women make informed decisions about family planning and birth control methods that align with their reproductive goals and health needs.

For women who wish to preserve their fertility for future pregnancies, preconception counseling may involve discussions about strategies to optimize fertility, such as timing of intercourse, ovulation tracking, and potential fertility preservation techniques such as cryopreservation of eggs or embryos. These discussions empower women to make informed choices about their reproductive health and take proactive steps to preserve fertility if desired.

Ultimately, the goal of preconception counseling is to empower women with CKD to make informed decisions about pregnancy and family planning, while also providing them with the necessary support and resources to optimize their health and minimize potential risks during pregnancy. By addressing medical, lifestyle, and reproductive factors before conception, healthcare providers can help ensure the best possible outcomes for both mother and baby.

3. Pregnancy Management: The management of pregnancy in women with Chronic Kidney Disease (CKD) requires a comprehensive and meticulous approach aimed at optimizing maternal and fetal health while mitigating potential risks and complications. Central to this process is the diligent monitoring of key parameters such as kidney function, blood pressure levels, proteinuria, and fetal growth throughout the duration of pregnancy. By closely tracking these indicators and adjusting treatment plans accordingly, healthcare providers can tailor interventions to address the specific needs of each patient and promote favorable outcomes for both mother and baby.

One of the primary focuses of pregnancy management in women with CKD is the ongoing assessment of kidney function, as changes in renal status can have significant implications for maternal health and pregnancy outcomes. Regular monitoring of serum creatinine levels, estimated glomerular filtration rate (eGFR), and urinary protein excretion enables healthcare providers to detect any deterioration in renal function promptly and implement appropriate interventions to mitigate further decline.

In addition to kidney function, blood pressure control plays a crucial role in pregnancy management for women with CKD, as hypertension is a common complication that can exacerbate renal damage and increase the risk of adverse outcomes for both mother and baby. Implementing strict blood pressure monitoring protocols and initiating antihypertensive therapy as needed are essential strategies for maintaining optimal blood pressure levels and minimizing the risk of complications such as preeclampsia and eclampsia.

Proteinuria, or the presence of protein in the urine, is another important parameter that requires close monitoring during pregnancy in women with CKD. Elevated levels of proteinuria can signify underlying renal dysfunction and may indicate an increased risk of adverse pregnancy outcomes, including preterm birth and fetal growth restriction. Regular assessment of urinary protein excretion allows healthcare providers to identify and address proteinuria promptly, thereby reducing the risk of complications and optimizing maternal and fetal health.

Fetal surveillance is also a critical component of pregnancy management in women with CKD, as the condition can impact fetal growth and development. Regular ultrasound examinations, fetal heart rate monitoring, and assessment of amniotic fluid levels enable healthcare providers to monitor fetal well-being and detect any signs of intrauterine growth restriction or other fetal abnormalities. In cases where fetal surveillance reveals concerns or abnormalities, appropriate interventions can be implemented to optimize fetal outcomes and ensure a safe delivery.

Overall, the management of pregnancy in women with CKD requires a multidisciplinary approach that integrates vigilant monitoring, tailored interventions, and ongoing communication between healthcare providers and patients. By addressing key parameters such as kidney function, blood pressure, proteinuria, and fetal growth, healthcare providers can minimize risks, optimize outcomes, and support the well-being of both mother and baby throughout the pregnancy journey.

In summary, special considerations in Chronic Kidney Disease encompass a diverse array of populations, including children and adolescents, older adults, and pregnant individuals. Tailoring approaches to diagnosis, treatment, and care is indispensable in addressing the unique needs and challenges encountered by each group. Collaborative efforts among healthcare providers, patient education initiatives, and robust support services are pivotal in optimizing outcomes and enriching the quality of life for individuals with CKD across all life stages.

10: FUTURE DIRECTIONS IN CHRONIC KIDNEY DISEASE MANAGEMENT

As our comprehension of Chronic Kidney Disease (CKD) progresses, so does the evolution of strategies and approaches to its management. This chapter delves into the forthcoming directions in CKD management, encompassing emerging therapies and technologies, promising research areas, and the significance of advocacy and community engagement.

Emerging Therapies and Technologies:

1. Precision Medicine: The evolution of precision medicine represents a significant paradigm shift in the management of Chronic Kidney Disease

(CKD), ushering in a new era of personalized approaches tailored to the unique characteristics and needs of individual patients. This transformative approach harnesses the power of genetic, molecular, and clinical data to inform customized treatment strategies that optimize therapeutic efficacy while minimizing the risk of adverse effects.

At its core, precision medicine seeks to revolutionize CKD management by moving away from a one-size-fits-all approach towards a more nuanced and individualized treatment paradigm. By leveraging cutting-edge technologies and analytical techniques, healthcare providers can gain unprecedented insights into the underlying molecular mechanisms and genetic factors driving CKD progression in each patient.

Central to the concept of precision medicine is the utilization of genetic and molecular data to identify key biomarkers and molecular pathways associated with CKD pathogenesis. By analyzing the genetic profile of patients and assessing molecular signatures indicative of disease severity and progression, healthcare providers can tailor treatment plans to target specific molecular targets and pathways implicated in CKD pathophysiology.

In addition to genetic and molecular profiling, precision medicine incorporates a comprehensive assessment of clinical data, including demographic factors, comorbidities, and lifestyle factors, to develop a holistic understanding of each patient's unique disease profile. This integrated approach enables healthcare providers to identify patient-specific risk factors, prognostic indicators, and treatment response predictors, guiding the selection of personalized interventions that address the individual needs and preferences of each patient.

One of the key promises of precision medicine in CKD management lies in the development of targeted therapies that directly modulate disease-relevant pathways and mechanisms. By matching patients with therapies based on their specific genetic and molecular profiles, healthcare providers can optimize treatment efficacy while minimizing the risk of adverse effects associated with conventional therapies.

Moreover, precision medicine holds the potential to revolutionize clinical trial design and drug development efforts in the field of CKD. By stratifying patients based on their molecular subtypes and disease profiles, researchers can design more efficient and targeted clinical trials that identify patient populations most likely to benefit from novel therapeutic interventions.

In summary, the advent of precision medicine heralds a new era of personalized approaches to CKD management, offering unprecedented opportunities to tailor treatments to the individual characteristics and needs of each patient. By integrating genetic, molecular, and clinical data, precision medicine holds the promise of transforming CKD treatment by providing more effective, targeted, and personalized interventions that improve patient outcomes and quality of life.

2. Regenerative Medicine: Regenerative medicine represents a groundbreaking frontier in the realm of Chronic Kidney Disease (CKD) management, offering tantalizing prospects for the restoration of impaired kidney function and the revitalization of damaged renal tissues. At the forefront of this burgeoning field are pioneering techniques such as stem cell therapy, tissue engineering, and organ regeneration, which hold immense promise as potential therapeutic modalities for CKD.

The overarching goal of regenerative medicine in CKD is to harness the innate reparative capacities of the body to regenerate functional kidney tissue and ameliorate renal dysfunction. Stem cell therapy, for instance, involves the transplantation of specialized cells capable of differentiating into various cell types, including renal progenitor cells with the potential to regenerate damaged nephrons and restore kidney function.

Similarly, tissue engineering approaches seek to leverage biomaterials and scaffold-based constructs to create bioengineered kidney tissues that mimic the structural and functional complexity of native renal tissue. By providing a supportive environment for cell growth and differentiation, tissue-engineered constructs hold promise for enhancing tissue regeneration and promoting renal repair in CKD patients.

Furthermore, the concept of organ regeneration involves the biofabrication of entire kidney structures using advanced 3D bioprinting techniques and cell-based therapies. By orchestrating the precise assembly of cells, biomaterials, and growth factors, researchers aim to create functional renal units capable of integrating seamlessly into the host's native kidney architecture and restoring renal function. Although regenerative medicine approaches for CKD are still in the experimental stages and face numerous technical and logistical challenges, they offer unprecedented opportunities for innovation and therapeutic advancement. Ongoing research efforts are focused on elucidating the underlying mechanisms of kidney regeneration, optimizing cell-based therapies, and refining tissue engineering strategies to overcome current limitations and enhance therapeutic efficacy.

Despite the inherent complexities and uncertainties associated with regenerative medicine, its potential to revolutionize CKD treatment paradigms cannot be overstated. By offering the prospect of functional tissue regeneration and restoration of renal function, regenerative medicine holds the promise of transforming the management landscape of CKD, providing hope for innovative and transformative therapies that may one day offer new avenues of treatment for patients grappling with this debilitating condition.

3. Wearable Devices and Remote Monitoring:
The integration of wearable devices and remote monitoring technologies represents a transformative shift in the landscape of Chronic Kidney Disease (CKD) management, offering a dynamic and patient-centric approach to healthcare delivery. These innovative technologies facilitate continuous, real-time tracking of critical health metrics, including vital signs, fluid status, and other relevant parameters, empowering individuals with CKD to actively engage in their own care and take proactive measures to safeguard their health and well-being.

At the core of wearable devices and remote monitoring technologies is the concept of patient empowerment, allowing individuals with CKD to assume a more active role in the management of their condition. By wearing these devices, patients gain access to valuable insights into their health status, enabling them to detect subtle changes or deviations from baseline more promptly and effectively. This early detection capability is particularly crucial in CKD, where timely intervention can mitigate the progression of complications and improve overall outcomes.

Moreover, remote monitoring technologies facilitate seamless communication and data exchange between patients and healthcare providers, bridging geographical barriers and enabling continuous care delivery irrespective of location. Through remote monitoring platforms, healthcare providers can remotely access and review patients' health data in real-time, allowing for proactive intervention and timely adjustments to treatment plans as needed. This real-time feedback loop enhances the precision and effectiveness of care delivery, leading to better outcomes for patients with CKD.

In addition to empowering patients and facilitating remote care delivery, wearable devices and remote monitoring technologies offer significant advantages in terms of healthcare resource utilization and cost efficiency. By enabling proactive monitoring and early intervention, these technologies can help prevent costly complications and hospitalizations, ultimately leading to substantial savings in healthcare expenditures. Furthermore, remote monitoring reduces the need for frequent in-person clinic visits, saving both patients and healthcare providers valuable time and resources.

The potential applications of wearable devices and remote monitoring technologies in CKD management are vast and multifaceted. Beyond tracking vital signs and fluid status, these technologies can also facilitate medication adherence, dietary monitoring, and lifestyle modifications, further enhancing the holistic management of CKD. Additionally, they offer opportunities for personalized medicine, allowing for tailored interventions based on individual health data and preferences.

As wearable devices and remote monitoring technologies continue to evolve and become increasingly sophisticated, their impact on CKD management is expected to grow exponentially. By empowering patients, enabling proactive care delivery, and optimizing healthcare resource utilization, these technologies have the potential to revolutionize the management of CKD, leading to better outcomes, improved quality of life, and reduced healthcare costs for individuals with this chronic condition.

Promising Research Areas

1. Biomarker Discovery: The exploration of biomarker discovery in Chronic Kidney Disease (CKD) represents a frontier of rapid advancement within the realm of research. This burgeoning field is dedicated to uncovering novel biomarkers that hold potential applications in the realms of CKD progression monitoring, prognostication, and treatment response assessment. Among the diverse array of biomarkers under investigation, urinary proteins, metabolites, and genetic markers stand out as promising candidates for facilitating early disease detection, predicting the trajectory of CKD progression, and evaluating the efficacy of therapeutic interventions.

The quest for novel biomarkers in CKD is driven by the pressing need for more accurate and reliable tools to enhance our understanding of disease pathogenesis and progression, ultimately leading to improved patient outcomes and quality of life. By elucidating the molecular signatures and biological processes associated with CKD, researchers aim to identify biomarkers that can serve as early indicators of disease onset, allowing for timely intervention and preventive measures to mitigate disease progression and complications. Furthermore, biomarkers hold immense potential as prognostic indicators, offering insights into the likely trajectory of CKD progression and the risk of adverse outcomes such as end-stage renal disease (ESRD) and cardiovascular events. By stratifying patients based on their biomarker profiles, healthcare providers can tailor treatment plans and interventions to align with individualized risk profiles, optimizing patient care and resource allocation.

Moreover, biomarkers play a pivotal role in the realm of personalized medicine, facilitating the identification of subpopulations of CKD patients who are most likely to benefit from specific therapeutic interventions. By identifying biomarkers associated with treatment response and drug efficacy, researchers can refine existing treatment algorithms and develop targeted therapies that offer maximal benefit with minimal risk of adverse effects.

The journey towards biomarker discovery in CKD is characterized by interdisciplinary collaboration and cutting-edge technological advancements, including high-throughput omics technologies, advanced imaging modalities, and bioinformatics approaches. These tools enable researchers to comprehensively interrogate the complex molecular landscape of CKD and uncover novel biomarkers with diagnostic, prognostic, and therapeutic potential.

Moving forward, the integration of biomarkers into clinical practice holds promise for revolutionizing the management of CKD by enabling precision medicine approaches that are tailored to the unique needs and characteristics of individual patients. By harnessing the power of biomarker-driven insights, healthcare providers can optimize disease management strategies, improve patient outcomes, and ultimately transform the landscape of CKD care.

2. Immunotherapy: Immunotherapy, a burgeoning field in the realm of medical science, is gaining traction as a potential therapeutic avenue for Chronic Kidney Disease (CKD). This innovative approach leverages the body's immune system to selectively target and eliminate detrimental cells, offering new possibilities for mitigating CKD progression and preserving renal function. By orchestrating immune responses and dampening inflammatory processes, immunotherapy holds the potential to attenuate the relentless march of CKD, thereby minimizing the burden of complications and enhancing patient outcomes.

The exploration of immunotherapy in CKD represents a paradigm shift in treatment strategies, moving beyond conventional approaches focused solely on symptom management towards interventions that address the underlying pathophysiological mechanisms driving disease progression. At its core, immunotherapy aims to harness the intricate interplay between the immune system and renal tissue, capitalizing on the body's innate ability to recognize and eliminate harmful entities while preserving the integrity of healthy cells and tissues.

Central to the promise of immunotherapy in CKD is the identification and development of immunomodulatory agents capable of selectively modulating immune responses to target disease-specific pathways and processes. These agents may include monoclonal antibodies, cytokine inhibitors, and other biologic agents designed to fine-tune the immune system's activity and restore immune homeostasis in the context of CKD.

Furthermore, research efforts are underway to explore the potential of immune checkpoint inhibitors, a class of immunotherapeutic agents that unleash the body's immune response by blocking inhibitory signals that dampen immune activity. By unleashing the full potential of the immune system, immune checkpoint inhibitors have the potential to unleash potent antitumor responses and may hold promise as adjunctive therapies for CKD.

Beyond pharmacological interventions, immunotherapy encompasses a broad spectrum of approaches aimed at harnessing the body's immune system to combat CKD. These may include adoptive cell therapy, which involves infusing patients with engineered immune cells capable of targeting and destroying diseased tissues, as well as vaccination strategies designed to stimulate specific immune responses against CKD-associated antigens.

While the field of immunotherapy in CKD is still in its infancy, ongoing research efforts hold promise for the development of novel treatments that target the underlying immunological dysregulation driving CKD progression. By unraveling the intricate complexities of the immune response in CKD and identifying therapeutic targets amenable to immunomodulation, researchers aim to usher in a new era of precision medicine tailored to the unique needs and characteristics of individual CKD patients. Through collaborative research endeavors and interdisciplinary approaches, the potential of immunotherapy to revolutionize CKD treatment paradigms and improve patient outcomes remains a beacon of hope for the future of renal medicine.

3. Artificial Intelligence and Machine Learning: The integration of artificial intelligence (AI) and machine learning (ML) technologies represents a transformative frontier in the landscape of Chronic Kidney Disease (CKD) management, offering unprecedented opportunities to leverage vast datasets, uncover intricate patterns, and forecast disease trajectories. Through sophisticated algorithms and advanced computational techniques, AI-driven systems have the potential to revolutionize various facets of CKD care delivery, ranging from diagnosis and prognostication to treatment optimization and outcome prediction.

At its core, AI and ML hold immense promise for enhancing the accuracy and efficiency of CKD diagnosis by analyzing multifaceted datasets encompassing clinical, laboratory, and imaging data. By discerning subtle nuances and identifying predictive biomarkers indicative of CKD onset and progression, AI-powered diagnostic tools can facilitate early detection and intervention, enabling timely implementation of preventive measures to mitigate disease progression and complications.

Furthermore, AI-driven predictive models offer valuable insights into patient-specific risk profiles and disease trajectories, empowering healthcare providers to tailor treatment strategies and interventions to align with individualized needs and preferences. By assimilating an array of patient characteristics, including demographic factors, comorbidities, and genetic predispositions, AI algorithms can generate personalized treatment algorithms that optimize therapeutic efficacy while minimizing adverse effects and treatment-related complications.

The potential applications of AI and ML in CKD management extend beyond diagnosis and treatment optimization to encompass prognostication and outcome prediction. By analyzing longitudinal data and tracking disease progression over time, AI-driven predictive models can forecast future clinical endpoints, such as progression to end-stage renal disease (ESRD) or the likelihood of cardiovascular events, enabling proactive risk mitigation and resource allocation.

Moreover, AI and ML technologies facilitate the identification of novel therapeutic targets and the development of precision medicine approaches tailored to the unique molecular profiles of individual CKD patients. By unraveling the intricate interplay between genetic predispositions, environmental factors, and disease pathogenesis, AI-driven platforms pave the way for the discovery of innovative therapies that target specific molecular pathways implicated in CKD progression.

As AI and ML technologies continue to evolve and mature, their integration into clinical practice holds promise for optimizing CKD management strategies, improving patient outcomes, and enhancing healthcare delivery efficiency. Through collaborative research endeavors and interdisciplinary collaborations, the transformative potential of AI and ML in CKD care remains a beacon of hope for realizing the vision of precision medicine tailored to the unique needs and characteristics of each CKD patient.

Advocacy and Community Engagement

1. Patient Advocacy: Patient advocacy organizations serve as pivotal pillars within the realm of Chronic Kidney Disease (CKD), undertaking multifaceted roles that encompass raising awareness, influencing policy reform, and fostering empowerment among individuals grappling with CKD-related challenges. These organizations serve as beacons of support, offering a spectrum of services ranging from educational initiatives and resource provision to community outreach efforts and policy advocacy endeavors.

At the heart of patient advocacy lies a commitment to amplifying the voices of individuals affected by CKD, advocating for their rights, and championing their needs within the broader healthcare landscape. By serving as conduits for patient perspectives and experiences, advocacy organizations facilitate dialogue between stakeholders, policymakers, and healthcare providers, driving substantive changes in CKD management and policy formulation.

One of the core functions of patient advocacy groups is to raise awareness about CKD, dispel misconceptions, and educate the public about the impact of the disease on individuals and communities. Through targeted outreach campaigns, educational seminars, and community events, these organizations strive to foster greater understanding and empathy towards CKD, thereby reducing stigma and promoting early detection and intervention.

In addition to raising awareness, patient advocacy organizations are instrumental in advocating for policy changes that promote equitable access to care, treatment options, and supportive services for individuals with CKD. By lobbying policymakers, drafting legislation, and mobilizing grassroots support, these organizations champion initiatives aimed at improving healthcare infrastructure, expanding insurance coverage, and enhancing affordability and accessibility of CKD-related services.

Furthermore, patient advocacy groups serve as lifelines for individuals and families affected by CKD, offering a range of support services tailored to their unique needs and circumstances. These may include peer support programs, counseling services, financial assistance initiatives, and navigation assistance to help individuals navigate the complexities of the healthcare system and access necessary resources and services.

Moreover, patient advocacy organizations play a pivotal role in driving research efforts and advancing scientific understanding of CKD through fundraising initiatives, grant funding, and community-based research collaborations. By mobilizing financial resources and fostering collaboration between researchers, clinicians, and patients, these organizations facilitate the development of innovative treatments, diagnostic tools, and supportive interventions that enhance CKD management and quality of life.

In essence, patient advocacy organizations serve as catalysts for positive change within the CKD community, leveraging collective voices and grassroots activism to drive tangible improvements in healthcare policy, service delivery, and patient outcomes. Through their tireless advocacy efforts, these organizations empower individuals affected by CKD, instill hope, and foster resilience in the face of adversity, ultimately shaping a brighter future for all those impacted by this chronic condition.

2. Community Engagement: Active engagement with local communities and stakeholders plays a pivotal role in addressing the multifaceted challenges associated with Chronic Kidney Disease (CKD), fostering early detection, prevention, and equitable access to care. Through collaborative efforts encompassing community-based initiatives, outreach endeavors, and educational campaigns, stakeholders unite to amplify awareness about CKD risk factors, symptoms, and available treatment modalities, empowering individuals to proactively safeguard their kidney health.

The foundation of community engagement lies in cultivating meaningful partnerships and fostering dialogue between diverse stakeholders, including community organizations, healthcare providers, policymakers, and individuals impacted by CKD. By harnessing the collective expertise, resources, and perspectives of these stakeholders, community-driven initiatives can effectively address the unique needs and challenges faced by local communities in the realm of CKD management and support.

Central to community engagement efforts is the development and implementation of tailored interventions that resonate with the cultural, linguistic, and socioeconomic diversity of the community. By adopting a culturally sensitive approach, stakeholders ensure that outreach programs, educational materials, and support services are accessible and relevant to individuals from diverse backgrounds, thereby promoting inclusivity and reducing disparities in CKD care delivery.

Community-based initiatives serve as catalysts for raising awareness, dispelling myths, and fostering a sense of empowerment among individuals at risk of or affected by CKD. Through targeted educational campaigns, health fairs, and screening events, stakeholders endeavor to empower community members with knowledge and resources to make informed decisions about their kidney health, thus promoting early detection, prevention, and timely intervention.

Moreover, community engagement extends beyond awareness-raising efforts to encompass advocacy for policy changes and systemic reforms that address the structural barriers hindering access to CKD care and support services. By advocating for healthcare policies that prioritize equity, affordability, and accessibility, stakeholders work collaboratively to dismantle systemic inequities and ensure that all individuals, regardless of background or socioeconomic status, have access to quality CKD care.

In essence, community engagement serves as a cornerstone of comprehensive CKD management and support, fostering collaboration, inclusivity, and empowerment within local communities. By leveraging the collective strengths and resources of diverse stakeholders, community-driven initiatives have the potential to affect meaningful change, promote health equity, and improve outcomes for individuals affected by CKD. Through sustained collaboration and collective action, we can create a more responsive, compassionate, and supportive ecosystem for CKD care and advocacy at the community level.

3. Research Collaboration: Research collaboration stands as a cornerstone in the pursuit of advancing knowledge and innovation in the field of Chronic Kidney Disease (CKD), forging vital connections among researchers, clinicians, industry partners, and patient advocacy groups. These collaborative endeavors, spanning multidisciplinary research consortia, collaborative networks, and public-private partnerships, serve as conduits for fostering synergistic interactions, pooling resources, and jointly addressing the complex challenges that underpin CKD management and care.

At the heart of research collaboration lies a shared commitment to accelerating progress and driving transformative change in CKD research and innovation. By cultivating a culture of openness, transparency, and mutual respect, collaborative initiatives empower stakeholders to transcend disciplinary boundaries, leverage complementary expertise, and tackle CKD-related issues from diverse vantage points, thus fostering innovative solutions and breakthrough discoveries.

One of the primary benefits of research collaboration lies in its capacity to facilitate knowledge sharing and exchange across diverse stakeholder groups, including researchers, clinicians, industry partners, and patient advocacy groups. Through collaborative platforms and knowledge-sharing forums, stakeholders engage in robust dialogue, disseminate best practices, and leverage collective insights to propel CKD research forward, catalyzing the translation of scientific discoveries into tangible clinical applications.

Moreover, research collaboration enables the pooling of resources, expertise, and infrastructure, amplifying the collective impact of individual stakeholders and maximizing the efficiency and effectiveness of research endeavors. By aligning complementary strengths and resources, collaborative initiatives can overcome barriers to innovation, accelerate the pace of discovery, and drive transformative advances in CKD diagnosis, treatment, and care.

In addition to advancing scientific knowledge and innovation, research collaboration fosters a culture of inclusivity and diversity, ensuring that a wide array of perspectives and experiences are represented in the research process. By engaging patients, caregivers, and community stakeholders as equal partners in the research enterprise, collaborative initiatives ensure that research priorities are aligned with the needs and preferences of those affected by CKD, thus enhancing the relevance and impact of research outcomes.

Furthermore, research collaboration facilitates the establishment of robust infrastructure and governance frameworks that support the ethical conduct of research, data sharing, and responsible innovation in CKD research. Through the development of standardized protocols, data sharing agreements, and ethical guidelines, collaborative initiatives promote transparency, rigor, and accountability in research practices, safeguarding the integrity and credibility of research findings.

In essence, research collaboration serves as a driving force for catalyzing innovation, accelerating progress, and improving outcomes in CKD research and care. By fostering collaboration and synergy across diverse stakeholder groups, collaborative initiatives harness the collective strengths and resources of the research community to address the complex challenges of CKD, ultimately paving the way for transformative advances that benefit individuals affected by this chronic condition.

In conclusion, the future of Chronic Kidney Disease management holds great promise, with emerging therapies, innovative technologies, and collaborative efforts driving progress in CKD research and care. By embracing precision medicine, regenerative therapies, wearable devices, and AI-driven algorithms, we can revolutionize CKD diagnosis, treatment, and monitoring. Investing in biomarker discovery, immunotherapy, and machine learning research holds potential for advancing personalized CKD care and improving patient outcomes. Additionally, advocacy, community engagement, and research collaboration are essential for addressing CKD disparities, raising awareness, and driving positive change in CKD management and policy. By embracing these future directions, we can work towards a future where CKD is more effectively managed, and individuals with CKD can enjoy better health and quality of life.

Vote of Thanks

Dear Readers,

I want to express my sincere gratitude to each of you for taking the time to read "Dealing With Chronic Kidney Disease: A Guidebook on Identification, Treatment, and Management of CKD." Your interest in this crucial subject highlights its importance and shows your dedication to addressing health challenges.

Your commitment to learning about chronic kidney disease is admirable. By exploring the contents of this ebook, you've demonstrated a readiness to equip yourselves with knowledge that can positively impact the lives of those dealing with this condition.

I genuinely hope that the information provided in these pages proves to be a valuable resource for you, whether you're a patient, caregiver, healthcare professional, or simply someone seeking to enhance your understanding of chronic kidney disease. May the insights gained from this handbook contribute to greater awareness, early detection, and enhanced management of this intricate condition.

Once again, thank you for your support and for championing health and wellness. Let's continue working together towards a future where chronic kidney disease is more comprehensively understood, effectively treated, and ultimately, prevented. Please feel free to give this book a good rating if it was helpful to you and comment on any other questions you feel should have been answered.

Warm regards,

Joshua Kendall

Printed in Great Britain
by Amazon